Kavita N Singh

Colposcopy Diagnosis Made Easy Quick And Accurate

Colposcopic assessment of the cervix using the modified Reid's Colposcopic Index scoring method

LAP LAMBERT Academic Publishing

Impressum/Imprint (nur für Deutschland/ only for Germany)
Bibliografische Information der Deutschen Nationalbibliothek: Die Deutsche Nationalbibliothek verzeichnet diese Publikation in der Deutschen Nationalbibliografie; detaillierte bibliografische Daten sind im Internet über http://dnb.d-nb.de abrufbar.
Alle in diesem Buch genannten Marken und Produktnamen unterliegen warenzeichen-, marken- oder patentrechtlichem Schutz bzw. sind Warenzeichen oder eingetragene Warenzeichen der jeweiligen Inhaber. Die Wiedergabe von Marken, Produktnamen, Gebrauchsnamen, Handelsnamen, Warenbezeichnungen u.s.w. in diesem Werk berechtigt auch ohne besondere Kennzeichnung nicht zu der Annahme, dass solche Namen im Sinne der Warenzeichen- und Markenschutzgesetzgebung als frei zu betrachten wären und daher von jedermann benutzt werden dürften.

Coverbild: www.ingimage.com

Verlag: LAP LAMBERT Academic Publishing GmbH & Co. KG
Dudweiler Landstr. 99, 66123 Saarbrücken, Deutschland
Telefon +49 681 3720-310, Telefax +49 681 3720-3109
Email: info@lap-publishing.com

Herstellung in Deutschland:
Schaltungsdienst Lange o.H.G., Berlin
Books on Demand GmbH, Norderstedt
Reha GmbH, Saarbrücken
Amazon Distribution GmbH, Leipzig
ISBN: 978-3-8433-6268-9

Imprint (only for USA, GB)
Bibliographic information published by the Deutsche Nationalbibliothek: The Deutsche Nationalbibliothek lists this publication in the Deutsche Nationalbibliografie; detailed bibliographic data are available in the Internet at http://dnb.d-nb.de.
Any brand names and product names mentioned in this book are subject to trademark, brand or patent protection and are trademarks or registered trademarks of their respective holders. The use of brand names, product names, common names, trade names, product descriptions etc. even without a particular marking in this works is in no way to be construed to mean that such names may be regarded as unrestricted in respect of trademark and brand protection legislation and could thus be used by anyone.

Cover image: www.ingimage.com

Publisher: LAP LAMBERT Academic Publishing GmbH & Co. KG
Dudweiler Landstr. 99, 66123 Saarbrücken, Germany
Phone +49 681 3720-310, Fax +49 681 3720-3109
Email: info@lap-publishing.com

Printed in the U.S.A.
Printed in the U.K. by (see last page)
ISBN: 978-3-8433-6268-9

Kavita N Singh

Colposcopy Diagnosis Made Easy Quick And Accurate

ACKNOWLEDGEMENT

With deepest sense of gratitude, I wish to express my heartfelt indebtness to everyone, who has helped me to take a step forward, in what always seemed to be an uphill task.

To begin with, I would like to thank my guide, Dr. Prof. S. Khare, for giving me opportunity to upgrade my learning in the field of gynaecologic oncology. Her constant encouragement, valuable suggestions and critical evaluation of my work, were guiding force behind this research.

I whole heartedly thank my co-guide Dr. Prof. Dhananjaya Sharma, who inspired me to think and execute new ideas in the field of clinical medical research. His optimistic criticism in research writing with prompt help and guidance were a boost to my enthusiasm.

I am grateful to Dr. M. Sant. And Dr. Savita Verma for cyto-pathological evaluation, discussion with them gave me a better understanding of pathological aspect of my research work.

I am thankful to Dr. Tapas Chakma for valuable help in study design and analysis.

I express my thanks to Dr. Prof. A. Lele, and postgraduates for there time to time support.

I acknowledge, Mr. A. Kavishwar for statistical analysis. I thank, Mr. Shailendra Koshta for typing and compilation of the thesis.

My family has been great support to me. My heartfelt thanks to my parents, who tought me the lesson of 'Excellence through Ethics and Education' in life. Words fail to express my thanks for my husband Dr. Narendra Singh and children Shashank and Nehal, who were uncomplaining, unconditional supporters throughout.

I thank almighty God for everything.

Dr. Kavita N. Singh

DEDICATED TO

To my late mother-in-law Smt. Rampyari Devi Nim

And

my father late Shri. SPR Diwakar

'Your blessings are my strength'

CONTENTS

INTRODUCTION

Cervical cancer is the second most common cancer in women worldwide.[1] An estimated 371,000 new cases of cervical cancer are identified every year[2] and accounts for about 190,000 deaths annually.[3] Out of all cervical cancers seen in world about 86% are from the developing world[4] and majority of them present in advanced clinical stages, as there is lack of infrastructure for early detection. Despite considerable knowledge and understanding about prevention, early detection, early diagnosis and treatment of cervical cancer, it continues to be the most common cancer and cause for death amongst middle aged women in many countries of South Asia, Sub Saharan Africa and Latin America.[5] In India it is estimated that there are about 126,000 new cases and 70,500 deaths due to cancer cervix every year.[6] In the last five years (2000 to 2004) out of 2557 female genital cancers, registered at NSCB Medical College Cancer Hospital, Jabalpur, 84.1% are cases of cancer cervix.

Prevention of invasive cancer by early detection and treatment of cervical intraepithelial neoplasia (CIN) currently offers the most cost effective long-term strategy for cervical cancer control.[5] For control of cervical cancer, education of community creating awareness, mass cytological screening, visual screening, colposcopy, HPV testing and vaccination against HPV are important preventive strategies.

The traditional approach to cervical cancer screening is dependent on use of Papanicolaou smear as an independent test.[4] Despite widespread clinical acceptance and use of this test, cervical cancer remains the disease of prime importance.

To intensify the cervical screening much attention and concern have recently been focused on the addition of a complementary test to cytological screening. Colposcopies, Cervicography, HPV testing and Polar probe are important investigation procedures to overcome the limitations of cervical cytology. If any of these procedures, used in conjunction with Paps smear they can maximize the potential of cervical screening.

As a procedure colposcopy has been around since the 1920's when Hinselmann realized that smallest non-palpable cervical cancer can be detected under magnification, so in 1925 he invented colposcope. In traditional role, colposcopy is a diagnostic test; visual test may also be used as screening tool.

Important problems encountered in colposcopy, are inadequate expertise, interpretive difficulties and failure to follow standard diagnostic protocol.[7] Considerable lack of agreement in reporting cytologic finding is a well-known problem, and lack of agreement might be an even bigger problem in reporting colposcopic findings.[8]

While practicing colposcopy in out patient department we felt, that colposcopy in spite of its high sensitivity in detection of CIN lesions is not very popular amongst postgraduates and even in practicing general gynecologists. We tried to investigate this issue to find out reasons behind it.

First problem was found to be inter observer variability in conventional colposcopy. Every time at the end of colposcopy examination, there was some difference of opinion in final diagnosis. To over come this we started practising RCI scoring, in each and every case, this solved our problem to great extent, disagreement and discussion came to minimum.

The RCI (Reid's Colposcopic Index) is a colposcopic assessment by scoring system that correlates colposcopic impression with histologic severity. The primary objective for the colposcopist is to identify the most severe lesion on the cervix, and perform a colposopically directed biopsy.[9]

We found this scoring method useful, to predict lesions with accuracy and, to take directed biopsies. This scoring method can further be used for follow up of low-grade lesions, if site specification is made integral part of it. This helps in better understanding of the nature of that lesion and there by its management. Reid or any other researcher had not mentioned this.

Second limitation to routine conventional colposcopy was, the time taken to complete colposcopy record was more then the time required for making colposcopy diagnosis. In our set up after central out patient registration, women comes to gynaecology OPD, with OPD ticket in hand. Post graduates take relevant history, do per speculum examination, if there is presence of risk factor for cancer cervix, it is noted and then after taking Pap smear, women is sent to adjacent colposcopy room. There post graduates are supposed to rewrite demographic details in two page colposcopy record sheet, take consent, and subject women for examination, all findings are noted in colposcopy record sheet as well as again entered in colposcopy department record register. This procedure of record keeping took over 20-25 minutes extra, in a very busy and over burdened gynaecology OPD. This tedious protocol is usually practised, in other teaching hospitals also.

To over come these practical problems we started documenting colposcopy diagnosis in equation style. (Details in material and methods and discussion) in OPD tickets it self, no separate colposcopy record sheet was filled. This made our job very easy, economic, and time saving.

Excited and encouraged by our preliminary observations, of this method, we decide to do detail study on present hypothesis. This was aimed to minimize subjective variability and disagreements, to make use of RCI scoring index in follow up of low-grade lesions, and to make colposcopy record keeping economical and time saving. We feel in future this study could be of great help for upcoming gynecologist in there learning and practicing colposcopy, there by they can contribute more actively, in early detection of cancer cervix, particularly in low resource countries like India.

AIMS AND OBJECTIVES

1   To do colposcopy assessment by modified RCI scoring method and study its significance in follow up of low-grade CIN lesions.

2   To Study impact of new documentation style in making colposcopy record keeping economical and time saving for developing countries like India.

REVIEW OF LITERATURE

Cancer cervix has been considered a preventable cancer because it has a long preinvasive state, screening programmes are available and treatment of preinvasive lesion is effective.

Screening for cervical cancer is one of the most prevalent and successful public help measures, for the prevention of cancer.[3] The easy accessibility of the cervix to inspection, palpation and application of cytology and tissue sampling procedure have led to extensive screening program for early detection and treatment of cancer cervix.

The Cervix :

The cervix is the lower fibro muscular portion of the uterus, measures 3-4 centimeters (cm) in length and 2.5 cm in diameter; however, it varies in size and shape depending on age, parity and menstrual status of the woman.[10]

The lower half of the cervix, called the portio vaginalis, opens through an orifice called the **external os**. Ectocervix is most readily visible portion of the cervix and endocervix is largely invisible and lies proximal to the external os. Ectocervix is covered by a pink stratified squamous epithelium consisting of multiple layers of cells and reddish columnar epithelium consisting of single layer of cells which lines the endocervix. The intermediate and superficial cells layers of the squamous epithelium contain glycogen. The location of squamocolumnar junction in relation to the external os varies depending upon age, menstrual status, and other factors such as pregnancy and oral contraceptive use.

Ectropion refers to the eversion of the columnar epithelium onto the ectocervix, when the cervix grows rapidly and enlarges under the influence of estrogen, after menarche and in pregnancy.

Squamous metaplasia in the cervix refers to the physiological replacement of the everted columnar epithelium on the ectocervix by a newly formed squamous epithelium from subcolumnar reserve cells.

The region of cervix where squamous metaplasia occurs is referred to as the **transformation zone**. Identification of transformation zone is of great importance in colposcopy, as almost all manifestations of cervical carcinogenesis occur in this zone. As the squamous cells at the original squamocolumnar junction mature gradually, it is difficult to differentiate colposcopically where metaplasia ends and the mature squamous epithelium of the ectocervix begins. Helpful landmarks include endocervix gland openigs, or gland ostia, which are characterized by central reddened residual endocervix encircled by slightly raised whitened metaplasia, and nabothian cysts. The new squamocolumnar junction represent the area of the most active immature cell proliferation, it is a site that must be completely seen by the colposcopist to accurately access areas where high grade dyplasia potentially develops. Vascular changes can be seen in areas of metaplasia. The optimal magnification to identify vascular changes is x 12 to x 16 over the original cervix. In adults, transformation zone is approximately 6 to 8 mm around sharp new squamocolumnar junction, which is easily identify after application for 5% acetic acid.

Cervical Intraepithelial Neoplasia (CIN) :

Invasive cervical cancers are usually preceded by a long phase of preinvasive disease. This is characterized microscopically as spectrum of events progressing from cellular atypia to various grades of dysplasia or cervical intraepithelial neoplasia (CIN), before progression to invasive carcinoma.[10]

Cervical intraepithelial neoplasia refers to the histopathological description where cells showing varying degree of dysplasia replace part or whole thickness of the cervical epithelium. It is graded into three categories depending upon the proportion of the thickness of epithelium showing mature and differentiated cells. CIN-1 corresponds to mild dysplasia, CIN-2 to moderate dysplasia, and CIN-3 corresponded to both severe dysplasia and CIS.

In 1980s, the pathological changes like koilocytic or condylomatous atypia associated with human papilloma virus (HPV) infection were increasingly recognized. Koilocytes are atypical cells with a perinuclear cavitations or halo in the cytoplasm indicating the cytopathological changes due to HPV infection.

This led to two grades of disease low-grade CIN consistent with koilocytic atypia and CIN-1 lesions and high grade CIN comprising CIN-2 and CIN-3. The high-grade lesions were considered to be true precursor of invasive cancer (Richart 1990). In 1992, The Bethesda System (TBS) for cervical cytology was introduced.

Important feature of TBS was the introduction of the term squamous intraepithelial lesion (SIL) and a two-grade scheme, low-grade (LSIL) and high-grade HSIL lesion. LSIL comprise flat condylomatous (HPV) changes and low-grade CIN. HSIL encompasses CIN-2 and CIN-3.

TBS is also used to report histopathological findings. National Cancer Institute, USA, revised TBS in 2001 (AppendixD).[10]

Diagnosis and grading of CIN :

CIN has no specific symptom that may indicate its presence, however CIN may be suspected through cytological examination or colposcopy examination, final diagnosis of CIN is established by histopathological examination of a cervical punch biopsy or excision specimen. Cytological assessment of CIN, based on nuclear and cyto plasmic changes is often quite challenging.

Nuclear enlargement with variation in size and shape is a regular feature of all dysplastic cells. Hyperchromasia is another prominent feature. Mitotic figures and visible nucleoli are uncommon in cytological smears. Abnormal nuclei in superficial or intermediate cells indicate a low-grade CIN, whereas abnormality in nuclei of Para basal and basal cells indicates high grade CIN. Nuclear cyto plasmic ratio is one of the most important bases for assessing the grade of CIN. Increased ratios are associated with more severe degree of CIN. Experience of cytologist is critically important in final reporting.

In colposcopy examination CIN lesion are identified by application of 3-5% acetic acid or iodine negative on application of Lugol's iodine solution, as the CIN epithelium contains little amount of or no glycogen. In histopathological examination, features of CIN are dependent on differentiation, maturation and stratification of cells and nuclear abnormalities. In CIN-1 there is good maturation with minimal nuclear abnormalities and few mitotic figures, undifferentiated cells are confined to the deeper layers (lower third) of the epithelium. In CIN-2 dysplastic changes are restricted to the lower half or lower two, third of epithelium, with more marked epithelial abnormalities in CIN1.

In CIN-3, differentiation and stratification in totally absent or present only in the superficial quarter of the epithelium, nuclear abnormalities extend throughout the thickness of the epithelium; many mitotic figures have abnormal forms. In CIS, anaplastic cells replace entire thickness of epithelium.

A close interaction between cytologists, histopathologist and colposcopist improves reporting in all three disciplines.

Etiopathogenesis of CIN :

A number of risk factors that contribute to the development of cervical cancer are; infection with certain oncogenic types of human papillomaviruses (HPV), sexual intercourse at an early age, multiple sex partners, multiparity, long term oral contraceptives use tobacco smoking, low socioeconomic status, infection with Chlamydia trachomatis, micronutrient deficiency.

HPV types 16,18,31,33,35,39,45,51,52.56,58,59 and 68 are strongly associated with CIN and invasive cancer cervix. Out of these 75% of cervical cancer are infected by with type 16,18,31 or 45.[11] There is strong association between persistent oncogenic HPV infection and high risk of developing CIN. HPV infection is transmitted through sexual contact and the risk factors therefore are closely related to sexual behavior. In most women HPV infection is transient and clears up within 12-18 months. HPV infection reaches a peak about 20-30% among women aged 20-24 years with subsequent decline to approximately 3-10% among women aged over 30 years. Inoculation of HPV occurs at the site of micro trauma during intercourse with an infected person.[11]

HPV infection is believed to start in the basal cells or parabasal cells of metaplastic epithelium. If the infection persists, integration of viral genome into the host cellular genome may occur. The normal differentiation and maturation of the immature squamous metaplasia into the mature squamous metaplasia epithelium may be disrupted as a result of expression of E6/E7 oncoproteins and the loss of normal growth control. The early low-grade lesion may eventually involve the full thickness of the epithelium subsequently, the disease may traverse the basement membrane and become invasive cancer, extending to surrounding tissues and organs. The invasion may then affect blood and lymphatic vessels and the disease may spread to the lymph nodes and distant organs.

Adenocarcinoma insitu :

The precursor lesion that has been recognized to arise from the columnar epithelium is referred to as adenocarcinoma insitu (AIS). Here normal columnar epithelium is replaced by abnormal epithelium showing loss of polarity, increased cell size, increased nuclear size, nuclear hyperchromasia, mitotic activity, reduction of cytoplasmic mucin expression and cellular stratifications or piling. AIS may be subdivided into endocervical, endometroid, and intestinal and mixed cell types. The majority of AIS are found in the transformation zone. AIS may be associated with CIN of squamous epithelium in one to two-third of cases.[10]

Preclinical invasive cancer refers to early cervical cancer with minimal stromal invasion, often without any symptoms or clinical features. Colposcopy has an important role to play in the diagnosis of preclinical early invasive cancer.

Screening methods for diagnosis of dysplasia and early cervical cancer :

1   Cervical cytology; The Papanicolaou smear.

2.   Liquid based, Thin Layer cytology.

3.   Thin layer based computer assisted screening.

4.   Cervicography.

5   HPV testing – Hybrid capture 2 system, PCR Insitu Hybridization.

6.   Speculoscopy.

7.   Papsure (Papsmear and Speculoscopy)

8.   Truescan (Polarprobe)

9.   Microcolpohysteroscope.

10   VIA (Visual inspection with acetic acid).

11.   Digital imaging colposcopy.

12   Videocolpography.

13   Optical biopsy.

14   Colposcopy (Traditionally diagnostic method).

Cervical cytology :

George Papanicolaou, an anatomist, devised the first system of reporting cervical cytology results and based the classification on the degree of certainty that malignant cells were present.

In 1928, he published a report titled "New cancer diagnosis" and devised first system of cervical cytology results in 1954. The system included five classes. In 1968 a new system was created that was based on morphologic criteria. This system known as "descriptive" was embraced by the World Health Organization (WHO). In 1978, Richart introduced the concept of cervical intra epithelial neoplasia (CIN), which encompassed all the precancerous epithelial lesion of the uterine cervix. Although this system described histological not cytological changes, many used the terms inter changeably to describe both.

The current cytologic terminology Bethesda system (TBS) was the result of the work of an expert panel, which convened in 1988 under the auspices of National Cancer Institute, USA. TBS replaced three level of dysplasia and carcinoma insitu with two levels, low-grade squamous intraepithelial lesion (LSIL) and high-grade squamous intraepithelial lesion (HSIL). Further refinements were added to TBS in 1991 and in 2001.

Liquid based, Thin layer cytology :

Liquid based cytology has been shown to aid in reducing the proportion of ASCUS diagnosis, probably based on improvements in both the fixation and the quality of the slide. Liquid based, thin layer technology was developed to overcome the technical limitations of the conventional Pap smear. The conventional Pap smear developed the technology to specifically address the five major limitations posted; failure to capture the entire specimen obtained, inadequate fixation, random distribution of abnormal cells, obscuring elements, and technical variability in the quality of the smear.

Collecting cells directly into a liquid fixative addresses the first two limitations. Mechanical mixing of the cells follows, mixing the cells creates a homogenous sample in which abnormal cells, if present are evenly distributed throughout the sample, hence third limitation is taken care. The final two limitations are addressed in very different fashion by the products currently available. The Thin prep and The Autocyte prep. Both techniques result in consistent, thin layer preparations of epithelial cells that are depleted extraneous elements. Both products produce slides containing 50,000 to 75,000 cells per slide in circular areas. Despite the limitations of the current data, more than 500,000 subjects have been studied, with a preponderance of data indicating a significant benefit of liquid based cytology in these samples ranged from low of 6% to a high of 110% with Thin prep technology and a low of 3% to a high of 137% by Autocyte prep technology.[11]

Thin layer – Based computer assisted screening :

Computer assisted devices have been shown to reduce the incidence of false negative Pap tests when used in a quality control mode to re-screen cases with a diagnosis of "within normal limits". Although large clinical trials are needed, these early results offer great promise for an improvement in screening sensitivity while reducing human effort and time spent.

Cervicography :

Cervicography has been proposed as an adjunctive test that would increase the sensitivity and specificity of the Pap smear for detection of precancerous and invasive cervical lesions. In 1980, Adolf Stafl, a colposcopist and photographer at the medical college of Wisconsin, invented a diagnostic method called cervicography. Cervicography is a method of detecting cancer and other cervical abnormalities by projecting, a photographic image of the cervix onto a screen, where an expert reviewer from a distance of 3 feet evaluates it.[3]

Tawa et al performed the first large study of cervicography in 1988. A total of 3271 gynaecology patients between the age of 18 and 50 years were screened. Results indicated that 5.1 times more CIN lesions were detected by cervigrams than by the Pap smears. The technically defective rate of the cervicography cervical cancer screening system is less than 2%. Early studies reported a sensitivity of 89% to 92% for detection of high-grade precursor lesion or invasive disease but specificity was low.[11] In addition to being used as an adjunctive test, cervicography has been used as a valuable research tool, for chart documentation, for teaching colposcopy recognition skill, and in the testing and monitoring of colposcopic skills. Studies show that per dollar spent cervicography detects more CIN lesions than conventional cytology.

Human papillomavirus testing :

The human papillomavirus (HPV) are the largest known subgroup of papillomaviruses (small DNA tumor viruses) with more than 100 types. Some are carcinogenic, whereas the majority cause benign epithelial lesions.

HPV is difficult to culture, one or more of three nuclei acid-based tests have been used for detecting and typing HPV in specimens. The polymerase chain reaction, the Hybrid capture 2 system, and in situ hybridization.

It is now widely recognized that HPV causes essentially all cervical cancers worldwide. Hence it may be agreed that HPV is an excellent marker of women at risk for neoplasia.

The median sensitivity of HPV testing for women with CIN-2 or CIN-3 and invasive disease was 93%, compared with 75% for the conventional Pap smear.[11]

HPV testing does not appear to be beneficial in young women, who are known to have predominantly transient HPV infection. The most compelling data for clinical utility of HPV- DNA testing in patients management relates to women with ASCUS Pap smear. Colposcopicaly CIN-1 and HPV is difficult to differentiate[12], but in high risk HPV colposcopy as sensitive as cytology.[13]

Speculoscopy :

Speculoscopy visualizes the cervix with blue white chemiluminescent illumination and low power, portable magnification following the application of dilute acetic acid.

A positive speculoscopy result is defined as the presence of at least one aceto white lesion that appears bright and distinct with at least one sharply marginated border on the cervix or vagina. Colposcopy is a more sensitive test than Speculoscopy.[11]

Papsure :

Papsure is a combine visual and cytologic test, which is considered positive when either the speculoscopy results or the cytology result is abnormal, and it is negative when both results are normal.

The negative predictive value of the combined speculoscopy and Pap smear (Papsure) is more than 99% and provides the option of widened screening intervals in women who test negative. Yu BK, Kuo from Taiwan, suggested that Paps and speculoscopy should be combined, as it is cost effective and accurate, he reported 92.9% sensitivity of Papsure.[14]

True scan (Polarprobe) :

The True scan (Polarprobe) device employs a real time approach to the detection of tissue abnormalities.

The device includes a pen shaped hand piece that is connected by a cable to a console containing a microprocessor control module and a digital signal processor. The hand piece makes contact with the cervix, ending low-level electrical pulses and optical signals.

True Scan has significant better sensitivity up to 97.6% and a lower false positive rate than does repeat cytology. Women experience less pain, bleeding and anxiety with True Scan than with the Pap smear.[11]

Microcolpohysteroscope   :

It enables in vivo examination of SCJ and endocervical canal with supravital staining at 20x, 60x and 150x magnification and provides cellular and nuclear details rivaling routine histopaholgy examination. It is particularly useful in evaluation of patients with discrepancy in cytology and colposcopy. It can also measure length of endocervical canal during conization.[15]

VIA :

Visual inspection with acetic acid is of interest to developing countries as it is inexpensive, only requires supplies usually locally obtainable, and can be competently performed by non-physicians with proper training. VIA has similar sensitivity to that of cervical cytology in detecting pre-invasive lesion but has lower as specificity.[16] As dependent and difficult to maintain quality control.

Digital imaging colposcopy :

The computerized digital imaging colposcope allows storage enhancement, and manipulation of a colposcopic image, serial observations, analysis and accurate measurement of lesion.[15]

Videocolpography :

Video colpography is an accurate, portable and quick method of cervical imaging. It combines the simplicity of a video camera with the versatility of computerized digital imaging and has great potential in the fields of teaching; audit and screening of low-grade smear abnormalities.[17]

Optical biopsy :

This process is based on the measurement of light-tissue interaction, which are analyzed by various mathematical and data processing methods, to provide information on the metabolism and morphology of epithelial tissue.[18]

Colposcopy :

Colposcopy is an optical method for visualizing lower female genital tract, under bright illumination at a magnification between the naked eye examination, and lower power of the microscope. It provides the study of surface epithelium, and the underlying stroma along with its vascular network.

As procedure colposcopy has been around since the 1920's. Hans Hinselmann assistant of a german physician Vonfranque, was assigned to study leukoplakias of the cervix that were observed with the unaided eye in many small cancers. Hinselmann expected to find a tiny focus of invasive cancer. He realized that in order to detect the smallest non-palpable cervical cancer, some form of magnification was needed to detect the smallest leukoplakia, and so in 1925 he invented the colposcope.

Chronology of early developments[7] :

1924   Hinselmann (Germany), preparing to revise a chapter on the cause, symptoms, and diagnosis of uterine cancer and studying the literature, decides that every clinical cancer of cervix starts out as small tumors or ulcers that might be detected using magnification and illumination.

1925   Hinselmann, develops a binocular microscope on a movable stand, including illumination, and conducts studies of the vulva, vagina and cervix, initiating the first colopscopy clinic.

1926   Babes (Rumania) introduces cytologic sampling of the cervix for the diagnosis of cancer.

1928   Schiller test was invented; Papanicolaou presents his observations of vaginal smear.

1929   Levy (United States) expresses the need for magnification, to study the lower genital tract.

1931   Emmert (United States) introduce the colposcope to North America with a Journal of The American Medical Association article.

1932   Colopsocpy used in a few centers in United States; Jacob (Argentina) visits Hinselmann and returns to establish the first colposcopy clinic in his country.

1933   Hinselmann publishes an introduction to colposcopy, describes a mosaic pattern.

1934   Sacks (United States) complains about cumbersome equipment, de Morales introduces colposcopy in Brazil.

1935   Unsandizaga (Spain) influenced by Hinselmann, refers to colposcopy in his thesis; Hinselmann estimates that the transit time from preinvasive. To invasive stages of cervical cancer is 10-15 years.

1936   Shaw (England) acquires a colposcope and begins colposcopy in England; photography of the cervix introduced by Creer and Bruner (United States); Gellhorn (United States) acknowledges the importance of colposcopy but complains about the expense and clumsiness of the scope.

1938   Hinselmann develops acetic acid test; Farrar (United States) advises that skill in colposcopy takes time and patience to acquire; Galloway (United States) introduces zoom lens photography of the cervix.

1939   Kraatz (Germany) introduces the green filters; colposcopic practice expands in Europe especially in Jena, Berlin,Zurich and South America, but war intervenes in European development; Papanicolaou and Trout (United States) begin working together.)

The second distinctive phase :

1940   Kranzfield (Switzerland) adapts the terminology used in gynecologic oncology reporting on Hinselmann's facilitating the adoption of colposcopy in Zurich, Rieper (Brazil) visits Hinselmann and returns to begin teaching; Hinselmann introduces the mercury lamp.

1941   Usandizaga (Spain) mentions colposcopy in paper on cervisitis and shortly after, Alba (spain) completes his doctoral thesis devoted entirely to colposcopy; Mueller (Switzerland) suggests the term stage for carcinoma in situ of the cervix; papanicolaou and Traut publish early findings of the cancer cells.

1942   Treite (Germany) produces photographs of the Cervix.

1943   Papanicolaou and Traut publish their book on cancer diagnosis by vaginal smears; a colposcopist is Switzerland

and Australia begins to use colposcopy to localize abnormal areas suggested by cytology.

1944 The first scientific articles (written by De la Riva) appear in Spanish journals and describe the value of colposcopy in preventing cervical carcinoma; Cytology begins to be introduced to Europe.

1946 Mestwerdt (Switzerland) introduces the term microcarcinoma.

1947 Alba write about the value of colposcopic investigations; colposcopy proliferates in Spain especially because many of the leading gynecologists of the time had been trained over the years by Hinselmann in addition to the fact that they were knowledgeable about pathology; Ayre (Canada) introduces the spatula for sampling the cervix.

1948 Colopscopy is mentioned in a British textbook of gynecology by Shaw.

1949 Hinselmann visits South America; Mestwerdt (Switzerland) publishes an atlas of colposcopy; colposcopy is introduced during the 12th British congress of obstetrics and gynecology by Stachan (Wales) by address and in his paper of the same year.

The rise of modern colposcopy :

1950 Colposcopy is widely practiced in Germany, Austria, France, Italy, Hungary, Yugoslavia, and other European countries; Navratil (Austria), installs colposcopy as a routine technique; Ando and Masubuchi (Japan) begin colposcopic studies to be followed by Karihara and Harai; Hungary institutes colposcopy for mass screening (10 years a head of cytology).

1951   Karaeneff (Germany) first uses electronic flash to produce high definition images.

1952   Palmer introduces colposcopy to France; Cartier's department acquires its first scope; Meigs (US) asserts that colposcopy should follow inspection of the cervix, Shaw (England) proclaims colposcopy as one of the most important advances, Novak's (US) obstetric and gynecologic pathology text book states that any discussion of colposcopy technique or terminology would "scarcely be profitable".

1953   Coloposcopist in Europe began to compare cytology and colposcopy results.

1955   Mcleod and Reid declare colposcopy popular.

1956   Hinselmann experiments with videocolposcopy.

1958   Navratil and collegues demonstrate 99% accuracy in diagnosis of preclinical cancer using cytology and colposcopy together.

1959   Hinselmann died.

1960   Coppleson discusses the value of colposcopy in preclinical cervical cancer.

1962   Spain advances use and reporting of colposcopy.

1967   Richart, introduced term cervical intraepithelial neoplasia.

1971   British colposcopy group formed, Coppleson, Pixley, Reid publish the first edition of colposcopy text, and establish the importance of transformation zone.

1972   First World Congress of colposcopy and uterine cervical pathology and cytology organized in Argentina.

1973   Stafl further develops colposcopy terminology.

1975   Second World congress, held in (Graz) Austria.

1977   Cartier publishes his comprehensive atlas of colposcopy.

1981   Fourth World Congress held in England on colposcopy.

1983   Japanese colposcopy society founded.

1985   Reid R, introduces RCI to grade precancerous lesions.

1985   Fifth World Congress held in Ride Janeiro (Brazil).

1987   Canada forms its own colposcopy society.

1989   Sixth World Congress held in Rome (Italy)

1990   Depalo (Italy) publishes a manual of colposcopy.

1991   Stafl, publishes, an international terminology of colposcopy.

2004   Monsonego J, highlights value of colposcopy and HPV testing with high risk HPV in clinical practice.

Diagnostic problems and limitations of coloposcopy :

Diagnostic errors in colposcopy are mainly due to inadequate expertise, interpretive difficulties and failure to follow standard diagnostic protocol.[8]

Considerable lack of agreement in reporting cytologic finding is a well known problem and lack of agreement might be an even bigger problem in reporting colposcopic finding.[9]

To minimize interpretation difficulties and select most abnormal lesion to biopsy, systematic colposcopy assessment system were proposed by Burghardt, Coppelson, Kolstadt and Stafl. Certain colposcopic criteria that were thought to be associated with abnormalities, especially higher grade lesions like leukoplakia, acetowhite epithelium, punctation, mosaic and atypical vessels, were defined Squamous metaplasia, gland openings, islands of columnar epithelium and nabothian cysts were considered normal findings. On basic of these criteria, grading system were developed.

Rubin and Barbo colposcopic assessment system :

The key concept of the Rubin and barbo assessment method includes the dimensions of colour, vessel, border, and surface pattern, and also includes description for normal findings. Lesion is graded into, Normal Grade-1/HPV/CIN-1/LSIL, Grade-2/Moderate dysplasia/CIN-2/HSIL, Grade-3/ dysplasia/ CIN-3/HSIL/CIS and micro invasion, frank invasion.[11]

Burghardt's system :

Burghardts system was meant to apply to colposcopy used, as a screening test in all women, not just evaluate those with an abnormal cervical cytology report.

The atypical transformation zone (white epithelium) is characterized by the hallmark of transformation but differs from the normal transformation zone in one or more of the following features. Colour, border, response to acetic acid, appearance of gland openings, surface contour, extent or size, iodine up take appearance of blood vessels, keratinization, erosion and ulcers.[11]

Coppelson's two-class grading system (1993) :

In transformation zone an actowhite area is graded into two grades; grade I insignificant and grade II significant.[10]

Reid's colposcopic index (1985) :

The RCI (Reid's Colposcopic Index) is a colposcopic assessment by scoring system that correlates colposcpic impression with histologic severity (Appendix C). The Primary objective for the colposcopist is to identify the most severe lesion on the cervix and perform a colposcopically directed biopsy.[11]

Learning to differentiate benign features from low-grade and high-grade CIN has been shown to be a challenge. More experienced colposcopist recognize that normal squamous metaplasia, various grades of CIN, and some cervical cancer exhibit varying degree of acetowhite changes, with or without abnormal vessel patterns. However less experinced colposcopist may incorrectly tend to accept all areas that demonstrate either acetowhite change or abnormal surface vessel as foci of preinvasive or invasive disease.

In RCI, colposcopic signs i.e. margins, colour, vascular patterns and iodine staining is scored and graded into two objective categories, low-grade CIN-1 or high grade CIN-2 and CIN-3, combined into weighted index called RCI, these colposcopic features are more than 90% accurate in predicting histologic findings, because this grading system relies on critical analysis rather than on pattern recall. Hence this grading system greatly simplifies learning colposcopy and ensures that serious disease will not be missed, and trivial findings will not be over interpreted. RCI provides a score, less subjective measurement of lesion severity and provides the examiner with direction for the target biopsy from most severe area on the cervix (Appendix A).

In our study cervix was divided into four quadrants by an imaginary line passing through center from 12'O clock to 6'O clock and 9'O clock to 3'O clock. Examination of each quadrant was done in clockwise direction starting from right upper (RU) quadrant (Fig. 1). If a acetowhite reaction was seen in transformation zone i.e. visual inspection with acetic acid (VIA) and visual inspection with acetic acid under magnification (VIAM) was positive then margin, color, vessels, colposcopy signs were scored by Reid Colposcopic Index (RCI) scoring method[11] and recorded in equation style. (Ref. Methodology)

MATERIAL AND METHOD

Study design :

This was cross-sectional hospital based survey carried out in Department of Obstetrics and Gynaecology, NSCB Medical College, Jabalpur during 01/09/03 to 30/08/05 with following inclusion and exclusion criteria.

Sample size :

Sample size was calculated using Epi info 2003 statistical software where (N=16,000) i.e. total number of women attending gynaecology OPD, where expected frequency of the disease was presumed to be at least 10%. (Based on available secondary data) with 99% confidence level, a total of 235 patients were required. We added 10% as non-response and 20% lost in follow up. Thus giving a final sample size calculated was 310.

Inclusion criteria :

Patients with history of intermenstrual or post coital bleeding, abnormal cytology report, abnormal or excessive discharge per vaginum, recurrent urinary tract infection and recurrent sexually transmitted infections were included in the study.

Exclusion criteria :

Women with bleeding at the time of examination, clinical evidence of acute infection, pregnancy and puerperium, unsatisfactory colposcopy, obvious growth and unmarried women were excluded from the study.

Ethical clearance :

Institutional ethics committee of NSCB Medical College Jabalpur, India approved the study protocol.

Data collection :

During 01/09/03 to 30/08/05 a total of 355 patients were screened and included in the study. Informed consent was obtained from all the women. Relevant socioeconomic, obstetric, gynecological and medical history was obtained in a pre-tested semi structured proforma (Appendix A). Colposcopic examination was done as per classical colposcopy technique.[11] Under illumination, per speculum gross, naked eye findings were noted.

Pap smear was taken by moist cotton swab stick. Two sample were collected by gently rotating the stick 3600, one from ectocervix and other from endocervix, so as to obtain representative samples from endo and ectocervix. Absolute alcohol 95% was used to fix the smear. Cervix was cleaned with soaked saline swab.

Colposcope, (Model No. MV200 Atagogiken Company Ltd. Tokyo Japan) was focused and cervix visualized under low power to note the abnormal findings. Capillaries and surface blood vessels of cervix were examined with green filter. Freshly prepared 5% glacial acetic acid (Appendix B) was gently applied for one minute over the cervix to ensure appropriate acetowhite reaction. Transformation zone was defined both at distal and proximal ends (As mentioned in review of literature). If squamo-columnar junction not visualized completely than colposcopy was said to be unsatisfactory and women were subjected for endo cervical curettage in same sitting. In satisfactory colposcopy cervix was divided into four quadrants by an imaginary line passing through center from 12'O clock to 6'O clock and 9'O clock to 3'O clock. Examination of each quadrant was done in clockwise direction starting from right upper (RU) quadrant (Fig. 1). If an acetowhite reaction was seen in transformation zone, i.e. visual inspection with aceti acid under magnification (VIAM) was positive then margin, color, vessels, colposcopy signs were scored by Reid Colposcopic Index (RCI) scoring method[11] and recorded in equation style. In present modification terminology   RCI-1 is used in place of CIN-1, RCI-2, for CIN-2 and RCI-3 for CIN-3 and each quadrant is labeled as per its position. This is documented with RCI score in that particular quadrant. For example, an acetowhite lesion in right upper quadrant (RU) with RCI score 4 will be documented as RU-RCI-2, and if the lesion is extended in left upper quadrant, the equation will be recorded as RU-LU-RCI-2. In cases where RCI score was zero, which is suggestive of sub clinical papilloma infection (SPI) or squamous metaplasia biopsy was not done and women was called for follow up after 6 months. If RCI score was 1-2 or more then 'Baby Tischler Forceps' took colposcopic-guided biopsies from the site with highest score. Tissue was immediately transferred to vial containing 10% formaldehyde and was sent to histopathological examination and pressure was applied to the site to control bleeding. Women were counseled for follow up and genital hygiene. They were reviewed with cytology and histopathology report after two weeks. Cytology, colposcopy and histopathology report were compared and further management was done. Women with normal transformation zone were labeled as colposcoy negative and those with evidence of an acetowhite lesion in transformation zone were labeled as positive on colposcopy. Cytological analysis was done by Bethesda 2001 classification (Appendix D). In first 150 cases conventional colposcopy record form (Appendix E) was filled, in next 166 cases colposcopy diagnosis was recorded by modified RCI scoring method on OPD slip only. Report of Pap smear, colposcopy diagnosis and or report of cervical biopsy were documented on same OPD slip, to minimize paper work. The reference standard for final disease status was histology report or negative colposcopy.

Fig.-1 Diagrammatic presentation of simplified RCI scoring method

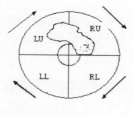

RU - Right Upper

RL - Right Lower

LL - Left Lower

LU - Left Upper

RU-LU-RCI-2

OBSERVATION AND RESULTS

A total of 355 women with high risk factors (history and /clinical examination) for cancer cervix were included in the study. During the study period 15,636 women attended gynaecology out patient department and out of them, 355 women were included in the study. Out of these 39 cases were excluded from the analysis due to missing/incomplete data. Analysis was a done with 316 cases. Pap smear was done in all 316 cases and cervical biopsy was indicated in 112 cases. Colposcopy was done in 316 cases and was unsatisfactory in 23 cases; in these cases endocervical curettage was done. In first 150 cases (group a) colposcopy diagnosis was recorded by conventional method and in next 166 cases (group b) by modified method. Follow up of low-grade lesion was done in 73 cases, after 6-8 months.

Table 1 shows distribution of study population according to demographic characteristics. The median age of the study population was observed at 35 years. In included group 56.6% of women were less than 35 years of age and 43.4% of women were above 35 years of age. In excluded group 51.3% women were below 35 years of age and 48.7% were above 35 years of age. The difference between included and excluded group was statistically not significant (P>0.05).

Table 1

Demographic characteristics of the study population

Characteristics		Cases Included n= 316 (%)	CasesExcluded n= 39 (%)	P value
Age	<35 years	179 (56.6)	20 (51.3)	P>0.05
	>35 years	137 (43.4)	19 (48.7)	
Locality	Urban	194 (61.4)	22 (56.4)	P>0.05
	Rural	122 (38.6)	17 (43.6)	
Marital Status	Married	304 (96.2)	35 (89.7)	P>0.05
	Widow	11 (3.5)	4 (10.3)	
	Divorced	1 (0.3)	0 (0.0)	
Education	Illiterate	149 (47.2)	23 (59.0)	
	Primary	109 (34.5)	9 (23.1)	
	Secondary	44 (13.9)	6 (15.4)	
	Graduate	14 (4.4)	1 (2.6)	
Religion	Hindu	279 (88.3)	35 (89.7)	
	Muslim	26 (8.2)	2 (5.1)	
	Sikh	6 (1.9)	0 (0.0)	
	Christian	5 (1.6)	2 (5.5)	

Table 2

Age wise distribution of the colposcopic diagnosis of the study population

Age group	RCI 1	RCI 2	RCI 3	Unsatisfactory	WNL	Total
<20	0	0	0	0	1	1
	(0.0)	(0.0)	(0.0)	(0.0)	(0.6)	(0.3)
20-29	17	8	2*	3	42*	72
	(23.6)	(11.1)	(2.7)	(4.1)	(58.3)	(22.8)
30-39	42	12	5	3	80	142
	(29.5)	(8.4)	(3.5)	(2.1)	(56.3)	(44.9)
40-49	13	10	11	9	37	80
	(16.24)	(12.5)	(3.7)	(11.2)	(46.2)	(25.3)
50 & above	5	1	3	8	4	21
	(23.8)	(1.2)	(3.7)	(10.0)	(5.0)	(6.6)
Total	77	31	21	23	164	316
	(24.3)	(9.8)	(6.6)	(7.2)	(51.8)	(100.0)
Mean	35.22	35.68	41.19*	46.04*	33.76	35.69
±SD	±7.87	±8.69	±10.75	±12.48	±6.86	±8.74

*RCI –1 Vs RCI-3 = *$P<0.05$(95% CI), RCI-3 Vs WNL = *$P<0.05$ (95%CI)

RCI= Reid Colposcopic Index

WNL = Within Normal Limit

Age profile distribution of colposcopy diagnosis of the study population is shown in table 2. A linear positive trend was observed as the proportion of RCI-3 cases is increasing with age. ($X2$ trend – $P<0.05$), Unsatisfactory colposcopies were more after the age of 40 years. 8 cases were suspected to have cancer cervix on colposcopy, were also scored as RCI-3, there mean age was 47.4±29.8 years.

Table 3
Distribution of presenting complaints of the study population

Complaints*	No. of Cases (n=316)	Percent
White discharge	310	98.1
Pain in abdomen	84	26.6
Itching perineum	46	14.6
Irregular menstruation	29	9.2
Burning micturition	12	3.8
No complaints	8	2.5
Post coital bleeding	7	2.2

* Multiple Response

Distribution of presenting complaints of study population is depicted in table 3. Majority (98.1%) of women. Presented with white discharge. Pain in abdomen was second common complaint 26.6%.

Table 4
Parity wise distribution of the study population

No. of children	No. of Cases	Percent
0	3	0.9
1	7	2.2
2	83	26.3
3	98	31.0
4	85	26.9
5	28	8.9
6	12	3.8
Total	316	100.0

Parity wise distribution of study population reflects that majority of women (84.2%) had two to four children (Table 4).

Table 5

Distribution of the study population according to history of contraceptive use

Contraceptives	No. of Cases	Percent
Tubal sterilization	186	58.9
Condom	6	1.9
Oral Contraceptive	2	0.6
Others	2	0.6
Non users	120	38.0
Total	316	100.0

Majority (58.9%) women had under gone tubal sterilization, 38% did not use any method of contraception, 1.9% used condoms and 0.6% used oral contraceptives (Table 5).

Table 6

Distribution of Per Speculum Observation in the study population

Per Speculum Observation	No. of Cases (n=316)	Percent
Ectropion	252	79.8
Infection	221	69.9
Hypertrophy	72	22.8
Healthy cervix	24	7.6
Nabothian Follicle	18	5.7
Old tear	9	2.8
Others	11	3.5

On per speculum examination, majority (79.8%) women had ectropion, 69.9% had clinical infection, in 22.8% women cervix was hypertrophied, healthy looking cervix was present in 7.6% and nabothian follicles were seen in 5.2% (Table 6).

Table – 7
Distribution of study population according to cytological reports

Cytological reports	No. of Cases	Percent
Negative for intra epithelial lesion (IEL)	265	83.9
Atypical squamous cell of undetermined significance (ASCUS)	15	4.7
Low grade squamous intra epithelial lesion (LSIL)	15	4.7
High grade squamous intra epithelial lesion (HSIL)	5	1.6
Squamous cell carcinoma(SCC)	4	1.3
Inadequate	12	3.8
Total	316	100.0

Distribution of study population according to cytological reports is shown in table 7 majority (83.9%) smears were negative for intra epithelial lesion, 4.7% of smears were ASCUS and LSIL, 1.6% smears were HSIL and 1.3% were positive for squamous cell carcinoma. (Out of 12 inadequate cervical smear 9 (75%) women agreed for repeat smear, out of them 7 (56.3%)were reported negative for IEL and 2 (16.6%) were reported as LSIL).

Table 8

Distribution of study population according to colposcopic diagnosis

Colposcopic Diagnosis	No. of Cases	Percent
RCI 1	77	24.4
RCI 2	31	9.8
RCI 3	21	6.6
Unsatisfactory	23	7.3
WNL	164	51.9
Total	316	100.0

According to colposcopic diagnosis the study population. 51.9% women were with normal colposcopic findings, 24.4% were diagnosed as RCI-1, 9.8% were RCI-2, 6.6% were RCI-3, and 7.3% were unsatisfactory colposcopies. RCI-1 includes 20 cases (6.3%) of HPVinfection, 9(2.8) cases of immature metaplasia, and48 cases (15.18) of CIN-1 (Table 8).

Table 9

Distribution of study population according to histopathological reports(HPR)

Histopathological reports	No. Of Cases	Percent
Cervical intraepithelial neoplasia- 1	12	10.7
Cervical intraepithelial neoplasia- 2	21	18.7
Cervical intraepithelial neoplasia- 3	2	1.7
Carcinoma in situ	5	4.4
Squamous cell carcinoma	8	7.1
Positive endocervical curettage	3	2.6
Chronic Cervicitis	52	46.4

Polyp	3	2.6
Inadequate	6	5.3
Total	112	100

In 204(64.6%) women with normal colposcopic finding cervical biopsy was not done, it was indicated in 112 cases (35.4%). CIN-1 was present in 10.7 %, CIN-2 18.7.% CIN –3 in 1.7% CIS in 4.2%, Sqaumous cell carcinoma in 7.1 %, Chronic cervicitis in 46.4%, endocervical curettage was positive for malignant cell in 2.6.% .

Table 10

Correlation between two age cohort and colposcopic diagnosis

Age cohort	RCI 1	RCI 2	RCI 3	Unsatisfactory	WNL	Total
<35 years	45	14	7*	4	109	179
	(25.1)	(1.8)	(3.9)	(2.2)	(60.8)	(56.6)
35 &	32	17	14*	19	55*	137
Above	(23.3)	(12.4)	(10.2)	(13.8)	(40.1)	(43.4)
Total	77	31	21	23	164	316
	(24.3)	(9.8)	(6.6)	(7.2)	(57.5)	

Out 316 cases 56.6% of women were less than 35 years of age and 43.3% women were more than 35years of age. Colposcopy was normal in 60.8% women of younger age group, where as in older age group colposcopy was normal in 40.1% of women. The proportion of RCI 3 cases above 35 years were more as compared to normal $p < 0.05$, (95% CI – 0.13 to 0.90) (Table 10).

Table 11

Distribution of colposcopic diagnosis according to duration of sexual exposure (in years)

Interval	RCI1	RCI2	RCI3	Unsatisfactory	WNL	Total
<10	8	7	1	2	26	44
	(10.40)	(22.60)	(4.80)	(8.70)	(15.90)	(13.90)
10-20	42	8	6	3	93	152
	(54.50)	(25.80)	(28.6)	(13.00)	(56.70)	(48.10)
20-30	21	14	10	9	39	93
	(27.30)	(45.20)	(47.6)	(39.10)	(23.80)	(29.40)
30-40.	4	1	2	4	6	17
	(5.20)	(3.20)	(9.50)	(17.40)	(3.70)	(5.40)
40 & Above	2	1	2	5	0	10
	(2.60)	(3.20)	(9.50)	(21.70)	(0.0)	(3.20)
Total	77	31	21	23	164	316
	(100.00)	(100.00)	(100.00)	(100.00)	(100.00)	(100.00)
Mean	19.03	19.38	24.90*	29.69	17.35*	19.36
±SD	±7.96	±8.74	±10.18	±12.77	±6.86	±8.77

Distribution of colposcopic diagnosis according to duration of sexual exposure in years in shown in table 11. Mean duration of sexual exposure among the RCI-3 cases was significantly more ($P>0.05$, 95% CI-0.10-0.77) as compared to those of normal colposcopic finding.

Table 12

Distribution of presenting complaints according to age group

Age group	White Discharge	Irregular menstruation	Post coital bleeding	Perineal Itching	Pain in abdomen	Burning micturition	No complains
<20	1	0	0	0	1	0	0
	(0.3)	(0.0)	(0.0)	(0.0)	(1.2)	(0.0)	(0.0)
20-29	69	2	3	20	8	7	1
	(22.3)	(6.9)	(42.9)	(44.4)	(9.6)	(63.6)	(25.0)
30-39	142	7	2	16	48	3	1
	(45.8)	(24.1)	(28.6)	(35.6)	(57.8)	(27.3)	(25.0)
40-49	78	16	1	9	25	0	1
	(25.2)	(55.2)	(14.3)	(20.0)	(30.1)	(0.0)	(25.0)
50 & above	20	4	1	0	1	1	1
	(6.5)	(13.8)	(14.3)	(0.0)	(1.2)	(9.1)	(25.0)
Total	310	29	7	45	83	11	4

Table 12 depicts distribution of presenting complaints according to age in study population. Between 22- 29 years of age, burning micturition (63.6%) and itching over perineum (44.4%) were chief complaints. Between 30-39 years of age, pain in lower abdomen (57.8%), excessive white discharge per vaginum (45.8%) and perineal itching 35.6% were chief complaints. Between 40-49 years of age 55.7% women presented with irregular menstruation and pain in lower abdomen (30.1%). Above 50 years of age 75% women were asymtopmatic.

Table 13

Distribution of colposcopic diagnosis according to marital status

Marital status	RCI-1	RCI-2	RCI-3	Unsatisfactory	WNL	Total
Married	75	29	20	20	160	304
	(24.7)	(9.5)	(6.6)	(6.6)	(52.6)	(96.2)
Widow	2	1	1	3	4	11
	(18.2)	(9.1)	(9.1)	(27.4)	(2.4)	(3.5)
Divorced	0	1	0	0	0	1
	(0.0)	(100.0)	(0.0)	(0.0)	(0.0)	(0.3)
Total	77	31	21	23	164	316
	(100.0)	(100.0)	(100.0)	(100.0)	(100.0)	(100.0)

Distribution of colposcopic diagnosis according to marital status is shown table 13 majority 96.2% women were married. Similar trend was observed in general population attending out patients gynaecology department.

Table 14
Distribution of colopscopic diagnosis according to religion

Religion	RCI-1	RCI-2	RCI-3	Unsatisfactory	WNL	Total
Hindu	66	26	18	20	149	279
	(23.7)	(9.3)	(6.5)	(1.2)	(53.4)	(88.3)
Muslim	8	2	3	3	10	26
	(30.8)	(7.7)	(11.5)	(11.5)	(38.5)	(8.2)
Sikh	3	1	0	0	2	6
	(50.0)	(16.7)	(0.0)	(0.0)	(33.3)	(1.9)
Christian	0	2	0	0	3	5
	(0.0)	(40.0)	(0.0)	(0.0)	(60.0)	(1.6)
Total	77	31	21	23	164	316

Majority 88.3% women were Hindu by religion, 8.2% were Muslim. 1.9 & Sikhs and 1.6% were Christians. Similar distribution is observed in general gynaecology outpatient attendance (Table 14).

Table 15
Distribution of colposcopic findings with multiparty

Parity	RCI1	RCI2	RCI3	Unsatisfactory	WNL	Total
Up to 2 children	22	8	2	6	55	93
	(28.60)	(25.80)	(9.50)	(26.10)	(33.50)	(29.40)
More than 2 children	55	23	19*	17	109	223
	(71.40)	(74.20)	(90.50)	(73.90)	(66.50)	(70.60)
Total	77	31	21	23	164	316
	(100.00)	(100.00)	(100.00)	(100.00)	(100.00)	(100.00)

(100.00)   Table 15 shows that proportion of RCI- 3 cases were significantly more (p<0.05, 95% CI-1.02 to 30.94) in women with more than 2 children as compared to women with less than 2 children.

Table 16

Distribution of colposcopic diagnosis according to complaints

Complaints	RCI 1	RCI 2	RCI 3	Unsatisfactory	WNL	Total
White	76	30	20	22	162	310
discharge	(24.5)	(9.7)	(6.5)	(7.1)	(52.3)	(98.1)
Irregular	5	3	5	2	14	29
bleeding	(17.2)	(10.3)	(17.2)	(6.8)	(48.2)	(9.2)
Post Coital	2	1	3	0	1	7
Bleeding	(28.5)	(14.2)	(42.8)	(0.0)	(14.2)	(2.2)
Perineal	16	6	1	2	20	45
Itching	(35.5)	(13.3)	(2.2)	(4.4)	(44.4)	(14.2)
Pain in	19	10	4	2	48	83
abdomen	(22.8	(12.0)	(4.8)	(2.4)	(57.83)	(26.3)
Burning	1	1	1	0	8	11
micturition	(9.0)	(9.0)	(9.0)	(0.0)	(72.7)	(3.5)
No	0	0	1	1	2	4
Complaint	(0.0)	(0.0)	(25.0)	(25.0)	(50.0)	(1.3)

Table 16 shows distribution of colposcopic diagnosis according to presenting complaints. In women with irregular bleeding 48.2% were normal on colposcopy and high-grade lesion were present in 27.5% (RCI-2 and 3). In women who presented with history of post coital bleeding 14.3% were normal on colposcopy and high-grade lesion was seen in 57.8% cases. In women who presented with itching over perineum 44.4% were normal on colposcopy. Women with complaint of excessive white discharge were as 52.3% and, were normal on colposcopy, 16.2% had high-grade lesion.

Table 17
Distribution of colposcopic diagnosis according to
per speculum observation

Per Speculum Findings	RCI 1	RCI 2	RCI 3	Unsatisfactory	WNL	Total
Ectropion	61	28	19	8	130	246
	(24.8)	(11.4)	(7.7)	(3.3)	(52.8)	
Healthy	3	2	0	5	14	24
	(12.5)	(8.3)	(0.0)	(20.8)	(58.3)	
Hypertrophied	11	3	4	4	22	44
	(25.0)	(6.8)	(9.1)	(9.1)	(50.0)	
Infection	56	23	13	11	114	217
	(25.8)	(10.6)	(6.0)	(5.1)	(52.5)	
Nabothian Follicle	40	0	0	0	5	9
	(44.4)	(0.0)	(0.0)	(0.0)	(55.6)	
Others	1	2	0	3	4	10
	(10.0)	(20.0)	(0.0)	(30.0)	(40.0)	

Ectropion was present in majority of women, and 52.8% of them were normal on colposcopy. Infection was second most commonest finding out of them 52.5% were normal in colposcopy. In healthy looking cervix 58.3% were normal on colposcopy 10.8% had RCI-1 and 2 lesion on colposcopy. (Which were mainly due to immature metaplasia or sub clinical HPV infection) (Table17).

Table 18

Quadrant wise distribution of the colposcopic diagnosis

Quadrants	RCI-1	RCI-2	RCI-3	Total
RU	35	10	2	47
	(74.4)	(21.2)	(4.2)	(36.4)
RL	16	3	0	19
	(84.2)	(15.7)	(0.0)	(14.7)
LL	10	5	4	19
	(52.6)	(26.3)	(21.1)	(14.7)
LU	14	5	4	23
	(60.8)	(21.2)	(17.3)	(17.8)
LL RL	0	3	3	6
	(0.0)	(50.0)	(50.0)	(4.6)
LU RU	1	4	3	8
	(12.5)	(50.0)	(37.5)	(6.2)
RU RL	1	1	1	3
	(33.3)	(33.3)	(33.3)	(2.3)
RU LU RL	0	0	3	3
	(0.0)	(0.0)	(100.0)	(2.3)
LU LL RL	0	0	1	1
	(0..0)	(0.0)	(100.0)	(0.7)
Total	77	31	21	129

*RU- Right upper, LU- left upper, LL- Left lower, RL-Right lower

Table 18 Shows quadrant wise distribution of the colposcopic diagnosis. Majority 83.7% lesions were present in one quadrant, 13.1% in two quadrants. 3.1% in 3 quadrants. Both upper quadrants together LURU had lesion in 65.9% women, and both lower quadrant together LL RL had lesion in 39.4%. Lesion were more in upper quadrant as compared to lower quadrant (t-3.022, df 128, P<0.01). Quadrant wise documentation of lesion helps in site specific management of high grade lesions and follow up of low grade lesions.

Table 19
Distribution of colposcopic diagnosis according to cytological reports

Cytological report	RCI 1	RCI 2	RCI 3	Unsatisfactory	WNL	Total
Negative for intra epithelial lesion (IEL)	63	24	6	15	157	265
	(81.9)	(77.4)	(28.5)	(65.2)	(95.2)	(83.9)
Atypical squamous cell of undetermined significance (ASCUS)	7	1	4	1	2	15
	(9.0)	(13.2)	(19.0)	(4.3)	(11.2)	(4.7)
Low grade squamous intra epithelial lesion (LSIL)	5	3	4	1	2	15
	(6.4)	(9.6)	(19.0)	(4.3)	(1.2)	(4.7)
High grade squamous intra epithelial lesion (HSIL)	0	1	2	2	0	5
	(0.0)	(3.2)	(9.5)	(8.6)	(0.0)	(1.6)
Squamous cell carcinoma (SCC)	1	0	3	0	0	4
	(1.2)	(0.0)	(14.2)	(0.0)	(0.0)	(1.3)
Inadequate		2	2	4	3	12
	(1.2)	(6.4)	(9.5)	(17.3)	(1.8)	(3.8)
Total	77	31	21	23	164	316
	(100.0)	(24.4)	(9.8)	(6.6)	(7.3)	(51.9)

Table 19 shows distribution of colposcopic diagnosis according to cytological reports. Out of 77 RCI-1 cases, majority 81.9% were negative for intra epithelial lesion 9% were reported as ASCUS, 6.4% as LSIL and 1.2% as inadequate. Out of 31 RCI-2 cases majority 77.4% smear were normal, 3.2% were ASCUS, 9.6% were LSIL, 3.2% were HSIL and 6.4% were inadequate. Out of 21 RCI-3 cases more than one fourth 28.5% smear were reported as normal, 19% as ASCUS, 19.0% as LSIL, 9.5% HSIL and inadequate. Out of 23 unsatisfactory colposcopies 65.2% were normal on cytology 4.3% were ASCUS, LSIL, 8.6% as HSIL and 17.3% as inadequate out of 164 normal colposcopies, cytology was normal in 95.7% cases, 1.2 % were ASCUS & LSIL, 1.8% as inadequate.

Table 20

Distribution of colposcopic diagnosis according to Histopathology results

Histopathology results	RCI 1	RCI 2	RC I3	Unsatisfactory	WNL	Total
Cervical intra epithelial neoplasia-1	6 (12.5)	5 (18.5)	0 (0.0)	1 (25.0)	0 (0.0)	12 (10.7)
Cervical intra epithelial neoplasia-2	5 (10.4)	11 (40.7)	5 (25.0)	0 (0.0)	0 (0.0)	21 (18.7)
Cervical intra epithelial neoplasia-3	0 (0.0)	0 (0.0)	2 (10..0)	0 (0.0)	0 (0.0)	2 (1.7)
Carcinoma in situ	0 (0.0)	1 (20.0)	4 (80.0)	0 (0.0)	0 (0.0)	5 (4.4)
Squamous cell carcinoma	0 (0.0)	0 (0.0)	8 (40.0)	0 (0.0)	0 (0.0)	8 (4.1)
Endo cervical curettage positive	0 (0.0)	0 (0.0)	0 (0.0)	3 (75.0)	0 (0.0)	3 (2.6)
Chronic cervicitis	33 (68.8)	10 (37.0)	1 (5.0)	0 (0.0)	8 (61.5)	52 (46.4)
Polyp	0 (0.0)	0 (0.0)	0 (0.0)	0 (0.0)	3 (23.0)	3 (2.6)
Inadequate	4 (8.3)	0 (0.0)	0 (0.0)	0 (0.0)	2 (15.3)	6 (5.3)
Total	48	27	20	4	13	112

Table 20 shows distribution of colposcopic diagnosis according to histopathology results. In RCI-1 cases, majority (68.8%) was reported as chronic cervicitis and 12.5% as CIN-1. In RCI-2 cases 40.7% were reported as CIN-2 and 37% as chronic cervicitis. In RCI-3 cases 70% were reported as CIN-3, carcinoma in situ, and squamous cell carcinoma. 25% were diagnosed as RCI-2 on colposcopy and in 5% chronic cervicitis.

Table 21
Distribution of presenting complaints in relation to cytology reports

Complaints	Negative IEL	ASCUS	LSIL	HSIL	SCC	Inadequate	Total
White discharge	260 (83.9)	14 (4.5)	15 (4.8)	5 (1.6)	4 (1.3)	12 (3.9)	310
Irregular menstruation	24 (72.7)	2 (6.1)	2 (6.1)	1 (3.0)	1 (3.0)	3 (9.1)	33
Post coital bleeding	4 (36.4)	1 (9.1)	3 (27.3)	1 (9.1)	1 (9.1)	1 (9.1)	11
Itching	47 (95.9)	0 (0.0)	2 (4.1)	0 (0.0)	0 (0.0)	0 (0.0)	49
Pain in abdomen	84 (89.4)	4 (4.3)	4 (4.3)	1 (1.1)	0 (0.0)	1 (1.1)	94
Burning micturition	19 (90.5)	1 (4.8)	0 (0.0)	1 (4.8)	0 (0.0)	0 (0.0)	1
No complaints	3 (75.0)	1 (25.0)	0 (0.0)	0 (0.0)	0 (0.0)	0 (0.0)	4

Table 21 shows distribution of presenting complaints in relation to there cytology reports 83.8% women with white discharge were reported negative for intra epithelial lesion. In 72.7% of women with irregular menstruation were negative for intraepithelial lesion. In post coital bleeding 36.4% were reported as negative for intra epithelial lesion, 89.4% of women with pain in abdomen with white discharge were reported negative for intra epithelial lesion. 90.5% women with burning micturition 95.9% women with itching over perineum 75%of asymptomatic were reported as negative for intra epithelial lesion. In post coital bleeding percentage of normal smear was lowest (36.4%) as compared to other presenting complaint.

Table 22 Shows distribution of histopatholgy reports with presenting complaints. Majority of women presented with excess white discharge in 71.8% of them were normal on colposcopy. Perineal itching, pain in abdomen and burning micturition had less little correlation with (CIN-1,CIN-2,CIN-3, CIS or SCC) histopathology reports. 57.2% cases with post coital bleeding (SCC,CIN-2), 17.2% with irregular menstruation(CIN-2,CIS,SCC) and 25% as asymptomatic(SCC), 11.0% with white discharge (CIN-2,CIN-3,CIS, SCC) were reported as high grade lesion on histopathlogy report.

Table 22

Distribution of histopathology results according to presenting complaints

Complaints	CIN 1	CIN 2	CIN3	CIS	Sq. Cell Ca	ECC	Inadequate	Polyp	Chronic Cervicitis	Bx not done	Total
White discharge	11 (3.5)	21 (6.6)	2 (0.6)	5 (1.6)	7 (2.2)	5 (1.6)	6 (1.9)	3 (0.9)	23 (7.3)	227 (71.8)	310
Irregular bleeding	2 (6.9)	4 (13.8)	0	1 (3.4)	3 (10.3)	0	0 (0.0)	3 (10.3)	1 (3.4)	15 (51.7)	29
Post coital bleeding	0 (0.0)	2 (28.6)	0	0 (0.0)	2 (28.6)	0	0 (0.0)	0 (0.0)	1 (14.3)	2 (28.6)	7
Perineal Itching	2 (4.4)	1 (2.2)	1 (2.2)	0	0 (0.0)	0	3 (6.7)	0 (0.0)	3 (6.7)	35 (77.8)	45
Pain in abdomen	3 (3.6)	6 (7.2)	1 (1.2)	0	1 (1.2)	0	2 (2.4)	0 (0.0)	6 (7.2)	64 (77.1)	83
Burning micturition	0 (0.0)	2 (18.2)	0	0	0 (0.0)	0	0 (0.0)	0 (0.0)	1 (9.1)	8 (72.7)	11
No complaints	0 (0.0)	0 (0.0)	0	0	1 (25.0)	0	0 (0.0)	0 (0.0)	0 (0.0)	3 (75.0)	4

Table 23

Distribution of Histopathology with cytology of the study population

HPR	Negative for IEL	ASCUS	LSIL	HSIL	SCC	Inadequate	Total
Chronic Cervicitis	46 (88.4)	2 (3.8)	3 (5.7)	0 (0.0)	0 (0.0)	1 (1.9)	52 (100.0)
CIN-1	9 (75.0)	0 (0.0)	2 (25.0)	0 (0.0)	0 (0.0	1 (8.3)	12 (100.0)
CIN-2	13 (61.9)	3 (14.3)	1 (4.7)	1 (4.7)	2 (9.5)	1 (4.7)	21 (100.0)
CIN-3	1 (50.0)	0 (0.0)	1 (50.0)	0 (0.0)	0 (0.0)	0 (0.0)	2 (100.0)
CIS	1 (20.0)	1 (20.0)	1 (20.0)	1 (20.0)	1 (20.0)	0 (0.0)	5 (100.0)
SCC	0 (0.0)	2 (25.0)	2 (25.0)	1 (12.5)	1 (12.5)	1 (12.5)	8 (100.0)
ECC	1 (33.3)	0 (0.0)	0 (0.0)	2 (66.6)	0 (0.0)	0 (0.0)	3 (100.0)
Polyp	2 (66.6)	0 (0.0)	0 (0.0)	0 (0.0)	0 (0.0)	1 (35.3)	3 (100.0)
Inadequate	5 (83.4)	1 (16.6)	0 (0.0)	0 (0.0)	0 (0.0)	0 (0.0)	6 (100.0)
Total	78 (69.6)	9 (8.0)	10 (8.9)	5 (4.4)	4 (3.5)	6 (5.3)	112 (100.0)

Considering histopathology as gold standard, cytology missed diagnosis of CIN-1 in 75% cases. CIN-2 in 61.9% cases, CIN-3 cases cytology was normal in 50.0% cases and CIS in 20% cases and none of the women was reported negative for IEL in SCC cases, this shows that cytology has poor sensitivity for CIN lesion as compared to SCC. Cytology underestimated diagnosis in 9.0% of CIN-2 cases, 50% of CIN-3 cases, 40% in CIS, and 50% in SCC cases (Table 23).

Table 24

Comparison of conventional and modified colposcopy method in relation with time required for colposcopy

Time (in minutes)	Conventional (group-a)	Modified (group-b)
<5	0	140
6-10	0	26
11-15	1	0
16-20	104	0
>20	45	0
Total	150	166
Mean	19.5	3.8*
±SD	±2.4	±1.8

* $p<0.0001$

Time required for colposcopy diagnosis and record keeping by conventional and modified method is shown in table 24. In (group -a) colposcopy was recorded by conventional method and mean time required in this group was 19.5±.2.4 minutes where as in (group-b) time required was significantly less 3.8±.1.8 minutes.

59

Table 25

Distribution follow-up results of RCI –1 Cases

Findings	No. of cases without biopsy (group-a)	No. of cases with biopsy (group-b)
Improved	16	15
	(55.1)	(34.0)
No change	10	18
	(34.4)	(40.9)
Advanced	0	7
	(0.0)	(15.9)
Lost	3	4
	(10.3)	(9.0)
Total	29	44
	(100.0)	(100.0)

* $p<0.05$

Out of total 77 RCI-1 cases, 29 of them, though diagnosed as RCI-1 but, as there score was zero biopsy was not taken (group a). In 48 cases RCI score was 1 or 2 hence biopsy was taken (group b), 4 had CIN-2 on histopathology report and were treated and 44 cases were advised follow up. From group-a 51.5% improved 34.4% showed no changes, none of them advanced and 10.3% lost for follow up.

In group b on follow up, 34.0% showed improvement, 40.9%% had shown no change and 15.9% of them advanced to CIN-2, 9% lost for follow up. All low-grade lesions (28 cases) with no change on follow up were treated by cryotharapy. 7 (9%) lesion, which were advanced to CIN-2, hysterectomy was done in 4 cases and LEEP in 3 cases. (Histopathology of these cases confirmed the CIN-2 diagnosis). Those improved from both groups were advised to come for follow up after 1 year.

Table 26

Distribution of colopscopy in relation to histopathology report

Colposcopic diagnosis	Histopathology		reportTotal
	Positive	Negative	
Positive	47 (51.6)	44 (48.4)	91(89.2)
	(100.0)	(80.0)	
Negative	0 (0.0)	11(100.0)	11(10.8)
	(0.0)	(20.0)	
Total	47 (46.1)	55 (53.9)	102(100.0)
	Sensitivity	100	
	Specificity	20	
	PPV	51.6	
	NPV	100	
	DA	56.9	

RCI-1, RCI-2, RCI-3 cases are colposcopy positive and CIN-1, CIN-2, CIN-3, CIS, SCC is taken as histopathology positive cases in calculation of sensitivity and specificity. Endocervical curettage revealed malignant cells in 3 cases but they are excluded from calculation, as in these cases colposcopy was unsatisfactory. Sensitivity of colposcopy was 100%, and specificity was 20%.

Table 27

Distribution of colopscopic diagnosis of RCl-2 and RCl-3
cases in relation to histopathology

Colposcopic diagnosis	Histopathology		reportTotal
	Positive	Negative	
Positive	36	11	47
	(76.6)	(23.4)	
	(100.0)	(50.0)	(81.0)
Negative	0	11	11
	(0.0)	(100.0)	
	(0.0)	(50.0)	(19.0)
Total	36	22	58
	(62.5)	(37.9)	(100.0)

Sensitivity	100
Specificity	50
PPV	76.6
NPV	100
DA	81

In high grade lesion (RCl-2 and 3) sensitivity of colposcopy was 100%, specificity was 50.0%, positive predictive value of 76.6%, negative predictive value was 100.0% and diagnostic accuracy was 81% (Table 27).

Table 28

Distribution of cytology in relation to histopathology report

Cytology report	Histopathology report		Total
	Positive	Negative	
Positive	22	5	27
	(81.5)	(18.5)	
	(46.8)	(9.8)	(27.6)
Negative	25	46	71
	(35.2)	(64.8)	
	(53.2)	(90.2)	(72.4)
Total	47	51	98
	(48.0)	(52.0)	(100.0)

Sensitivity	46.8
Specificity	90.2
PPV	81.5
NPV	64.8
DA	69.4

Sensitivity of cytology in detection of preinvasive cervical lesion was 46.8% specificity was 90.2%, positive predictive value was 81.5% negative predictive value was 64.8% and diagnostic accuracy was 69.4% (Table 28).

Table 29

Distribution of visual inspection with acetic acid in relation to histopathology report

Visual inspection with acetic acid	Histopathology report		Total
	Positive	Negative	
Positive	48 (58.5)	34 (41.5)	82
	(94.1)	(61.8)	(74.4)
Negative	3 (12.5)	21 (87.5)	24
	(5.9)	(38.2)	(22.6)
Total	51 (48.1)	55 (51.9)	106 (100.0)

Sensitivity 94.1

Specificity 38.2   PPV 58.5

NPV 87.5

Sensitivity of visual inspection with acetic acid in detection of preinvasive cervical lesion was 94.1% specificity was 38.2%, positive predictive value was 58.5% negative predictive value was 87.5%   (Table 29).

Table 30
Comparison of present study with other studies

		AHCPR (Based on 845 studies) 1999	N. Sundari Banglore 2000	Shashtri Mumbai 2005	J.L. Benedet Canada 2005	Kavita N Singh Jabalpur 2005
Colposcopy	Sensitivity	-	87.6%	75.4%	90.3%	100 (100.0%)*
	Specificity	-	43.4%	86.3%	57.7% (50.0%)*	20.0%
Cytology	Sensitivity	51%	57.7%	57.4%	-	46.8%
	Specificity	98%	82.6%	98.6%	-	90.2%

* High Grade Lesion

Table 30 shows comparison of present study with other studies. In present study, colposcopy sensitivity was 100.0% and specificity was 20.0%, where as in high-grade lesion was 50.0%. Cytology sensitivity was 46.8% and specificity was 90.2%.

Plate 1, Photograph of Colposcope used in this study

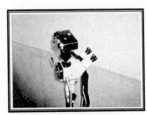

Colposcope With Camera
(Model No. MV 200 Atagogiken Co. Ltd.,Tokyo,Japan)

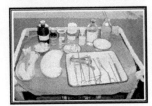

Colposcopy Instrument Tray

Plate 2 Showing Immature Metaplasia

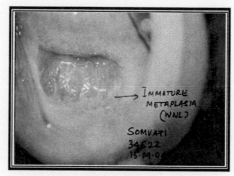

The "New" Squamocoluminar Junction With Immature Metaplasia

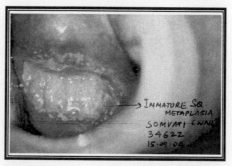

Partial Iodine Uptake by Immature Squamous Epithelium

Plate 3 Colposcopy Photographs

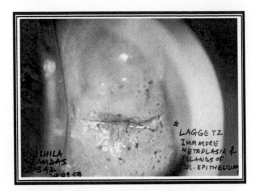

Large Transformation Zone With Immature Metaplasia
And Multiple Islands of Columinar Epithelium

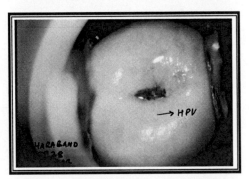

Geographic Satellite Low Grade Lesion (RLRCI-1)

Plate 4 Colposcopy Photographs

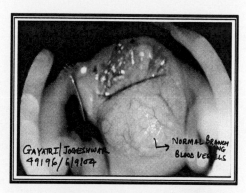

Prominent Normal Arborizing Vessels

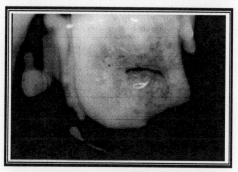

Abnormal Blood Vessels Examined With Green Filter
(Biopsy Suggestive Of Epidermoid Carcinoma)

Plate 5 Colposcopy Photographs

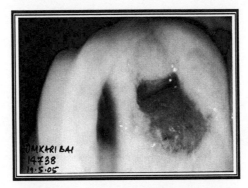

Transformation Zone After Application of Saline

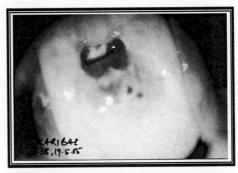

**Dense Acetowhite Lesion On Anterior Lip And Two Cuffed
Openings With Mild Acetowhite Lesion On Posterior Lip
Moderate Dysplasia (LURCI-2, RLRCI-1)**

Plate – 6 Colposcopy Photographs

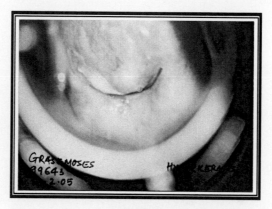

Leukoplakia
(Before Application of 5% Acetic Acid)

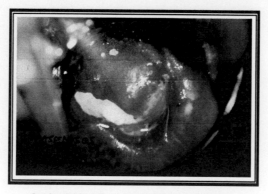

Leukoplakia After Lugol's Iodine Application

Plate 7 Colposcopy Photographs

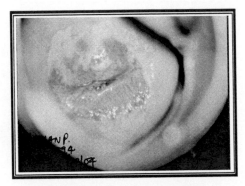

Intermediate Grade Lesion (LU,RLRCI-2)

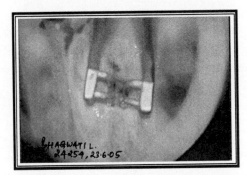

Visualization Of AW Lesion Its Extent In Endocervical Canal

Plate – 8 Colposcopy Photographs

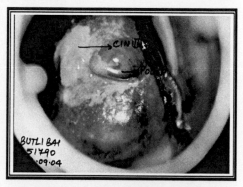

Rejection Of Iodine In High Grade Lesion
(LL-RL,RCI-3)

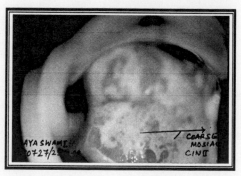

Mosiac With Dilated Punctation In High Grade Lesion
(LU-RURCI-3)

Plate – 9 Colposcopy Photographs

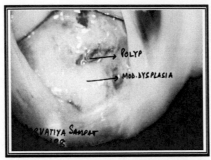

Polyp With Dense Aceto White Lesion (LU-LLRCI-2)

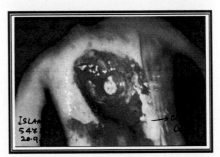

**Diffuse Dense White Lesion With Sharply Demarcated Margins
With Mosiac In High Grade Lesion**

DISCUSSION

The present prospective study was conducted in out patients department of obstetrics and gynaecology, NSCB Medical College during 01/09/03 to 30/08/05.

Cervical cancer is a significant reproductive health problem in developing world, hence cancer prevention or early detection becomes medico social responsibility and economic necessity.[19] Out of all cervical cancer cases seen in the world 14% occurs in the developed countries and about 86% occur in developing world, where as we know that cervical cancer is considered to be preventable disease (by WHO), as it can be diagnosed in its pre-cancerous phase and can be controlled.[3] Screening for cervical cancer is one of the most prevalent and successful public health measures for the prevention of cancer.[4] There are various methods for screening like conventional cytology i.e. Pap smear, thin layer cytology. Pap sure, speculoscopy, HPV testing, colposcopy, video colposcopy etc. Out of all screening methods, cervical cytology in the most widely used screening test. Conventional cytology has reduced the burden of cervical cancer in developed countries, however it is unsuccessful in reducing cervical cancer mortality in countries like India where, it is in operation for more than 30 years.

A critical appraisal of reason for the failure of suboptimal performance of cytology screening has led to the evaluation of alternative testing. The most dependable and best diagnostic methods for detection of cervical cancer may, of course be direct

75

inspection of the transformation zone of the cervix with the naked eye, collection of cytology material for, HPV-DNA test, colposcopy and guided biopsy or cervicography. Naked eye examination like VIA, VILI are simple and cheap method for down staging of cancer cervix in low resource setting, but has high false positive rates.

HPV-DNA test is a promising approach and is the most reproducible of all cervical screening test, but it is costlier (20-30 US $) than other screening tests, and requires sophisticated laboratory infrastructure including testing equipment, storage facilities for samples and trained technicians,[11] hence not an ideal method of screening for developing countries.

Cervicography was developed by Adolf Stafl in 1981 obtaining a quality cervicography picture and evaluation of slides is done by experts in colposcopy (Experience of at least 5 years), who have had additional training in the technique of evaluation of cervicography slides. Hence one should be colposcopy expert first than, can be cervicography expert.[11]

As a procedure colposcopy has been around since the 1920, when the colposcopy was little more than an inexpensive, optically modified binocular with an illuminator on the upper surface but today colposcopy is accepted worldwide as the most studied method for detection of early cervical cancer. In traditional role, colposcopy is a diagnostic test; visual test may also be used as screening tool. While performing colposcopy in day-to-day practice in our institution, we found several practical difficulties, as limitations.

1-   In conventional colposcopy interobeserver variability was significant problem, to over come; we started doing all colposcopic assessment by Reid's Colposcopy Index, which is a scoring system that correlates colposcopic impression with histological severity. This helped us significantly to increase predictive accuracy of lesion.

2-　　　In conventional colposcopy results are recorded by photographs and hand drawings, position of SCJ, TZ and various colposcopic patterns are also marked.

Buxton EJ. from UK, explained by applying a grid to the image of cervix creating eight sectors, (4 outer and 4 inner sectors) involved and findings recorded on proforma and graph.[20]

Odell's and Hammonds diagram is the simplest, of all existing documentation style. Hammonds graph has twelve sections divided by concentric circles to mark the findings at more precise site. Lesion can be specified using the abbreviations as in Odell's diagram.[8]

These methods are cheap but time consuming photographs are good, but quality and cost is limiting factor. In existing protocol, demographic forms, clinical findings with diagram, laboratory report of cytology and or histopathology, patients education card with follow up protocol is mandatory.[11]

We realized that time required in completing colposcopy record in outpatient department was three times more than the time required for colposcopy examination and interpretation. Colposcopy though being very sensitive method in early detection of cancer cervix is not popular among gynecologists of developing country like India, particularly tertiary care centers, where hospitals are overburdened and quick disposal of patients is absolute necessity. To reduce paper work without compromising accuracy in diagnosis, new equation style for documentation has been suggested. In our hypothesis, interpretation and documentation both are made easy. It greatly simplifies learning colposcopy and ensures that disease is not missed. **3-** Reid's colpocopy Index as described by Reid is useful to predict lesion with accuracy and take directed biopsies. Importance of site specification is not mentioned or suggested by Reid. In modified RCI scoring method equation style has site specification as integral part of it. This is very useful for follow up of low-grade lesions and site-specific management of these lesions. (Ref. Table 25)

Fig. -2

Modified RCI Scoring Method
Example with follow up figures)

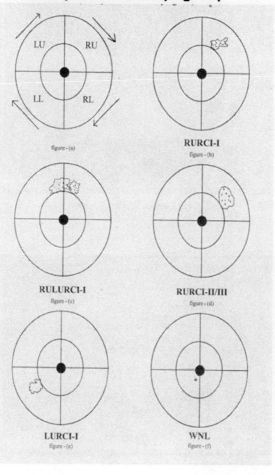

figure - (a)

RURCI-I
figure - (b)

RULURCI-I
figure - (c)

RURCI-II/III
figure - (d)

LURCI-I
figure - (e)

WNL
figure - (f)

Plate - 10 Colposcopy Photographs

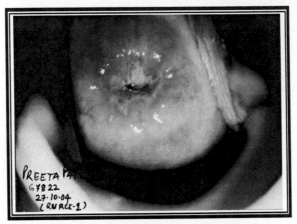

**Low Grade Lesion With Cytology LSIL
(RURCI-1)**

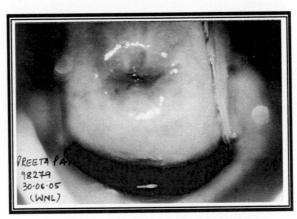

**Same Patient On Follow Up Colposcopy WNL And
Cytology Negative For Intra Epithelial Lesion**

Cervix was divided into four quadrants and examination was done in clock wise direction starting from right upper quadrant, each quadrant is scored and documented in equation style Fig-2 (figure-a). For example, If a patient has low-grade lesion in right upper quadrant of cervix, it will be documented as RU, RCI-1 (figure-b) and on follow up colposcopy if this patients comes to same colposcopist or goes to any other colopocopist, one can understand the grade of lesion on previous date of examination and can correlate with present examination findings.

For example (i) If same lesion extends to left upper lip of cervix also than it will be documented as RU,LURCI-1 (figure-c). (ii) If it has increased in severity at the same site than it will be documented as RURCI-2 (figure-d). (iii) If this low-grade lesion disappears and another low grade lesion appears in left lower quadrant than current equation will be LL,RCI-1 (figure-e). (iv) If in case lesion disappears completely (as often seen in HPV infections or mild dysplasia secondary to local infection), It will be documented RURCI-1 converted to within normal limits (figure-f).

Advantage of Modified RCI Scoring Method :

1 Colposcopy diagnosis was made, site specific hence very useful in follow up of low-grade lesions and quadrant wise site specific management (Table 18), **as seen in plate 10 RU RCI-1 is converted to WNL.**

2 As demographic information, history and clinical findings are already documented in outpatient ticket, if high risk factors present in history or clinical examination women were subjected for screening colposcopy preferably in same visit. Follow up advice and treatment was mentioned in same OPD ticket. Hence no extra visits, no extra paperwork, and time

81

taken was significantly less than conventional colposcopy (Table 24).

3   Inter observer variability was minimum as all lesion were scored by Reids Colposcopy Index.

4   This method is easy to train and teach colposcopy.

Other observations :

Majority of (70.2%) women were between 30-50 years, mean age of studied cases was 35.6± 8.74 years (Table 2). Similar observation was made by Sundari N.[21] and Bharani B. et al.[22]

About 61.4% women were from urban area and there mean age was lower than the rural population, which could be due to more awareness and better access to health care facilities in urban area than rural area (Table 1).

Mean age of cases diagnosed as cancer cervix was 47.42 ± 9.83 years and that of RCI-1, 2 & 3 was 35.22 ± 7.87 and 35.68 ± 8..69, 41.19 ± 10.75 years, a linear positive trend was observed as the proportion of RCI-3 cases, is increasing with the age   (Table 2) this clearly indicates that invasive carcinoma ivolves after a long period (10 Years or more) of preinvasive or intra epithelial neoplasia, and there are clearly two nodes of age where chances of positive non invasive and invasive lesion could be seen first around 35 years and second around 50 years of age.   Similar comment is quoted by, Bhatla N.

According to bulletin WHO meeting[24], risk of cancer cervix is 10 folds more with multiparity or if sexual activity begins before age of 15 years, similar observation was present in our study where, majority (96.9%) were multipara. Mean duration of sexual exposure in RCI-3 cases was significantly more (Table 11) CIN is most likely to begin at menarch or after pregnancy when metaplasia is most active. This could be due to active metaplasia during adolscence hence potential for interaction between carcinogen and cervix is increased.[25]

Majority 65.9% lesion were present on anterior up of cervix (Table 18), similar note is mentioned in Novak's Textbook of Gynaecology.[26] In studied cases 58.9% women underwent permanent sterilization operation and 38% women did not use any method of contraception, thus in total 96.9% women, no barrier method was used (Table 5) and 98.9% women were exposed to sex for duration between 10-40 years of there active reproductive life (Table 11). This strengthens the hypothesis that carcinogen are transmitted via coitus to exposed cervix.[25]

Low socio economic status, teenage marriage, multiparity, anemia, smoking, and tobacco use (active or passive) was found to be associated as co-risk factors, in our study. The single most

familiar screening test for detection of cancer cervix is Pap test, despite its unparalleled success, deficiencies exIst and these have been the target of numerous studies and new techniques within the past 5-7 years. Although designed to improve accuracy of Pap test, it is know that 100% accuracy is unachievable.[27]

On basis of 84 studies, the agency for Health Care Policy and Research reported that conventional cytology has a specificity of 98% and a sensitivity of 51%.[11] In adequate sampling and sample transfer by traditional methods are the major causes of false negative results, accounting for approximately 50% of missed significant lesion.

False negative rate of Pap test range from 6-55% due to sampling or diagnostic errors.[11] In some cases, cervical cancers are undetected despite a recent screening test because of errors in sampling, interpretation or follow up.

In our study cervical cytology showed 46.84% sensitivity and 90.2% specificity. Similar observations are made by others (Table 30). Agency for health care policy and research reported that conventional cytology has a specificity of 98% and sensitivity of 51%.[11]

Table 28 shows correlation of cytolgy with HPR, out of 98 eligible cases for analysis, 47(48.0%) were positive by HPR, out of these only 22(46.8%) cases were positive by cytology, thus sensitivity of cytology was 46.8% and specificity was 90.2% positive predictive value was 81.5% and negative predictive value was 64.8% diagnostic accuracy was 69.4%.

Shastri et al from TMH Mumbai, reported cytological sensitivity 57.4% and specificity 98.6%.[28] Yu BK, KuoBI, from Taiwan reported sensitivity of cytology 45.2%.[14] Sundari N. from Banglore reported false negative rate of 22.4%, sensitivity of 57.4% and specificity of 82.6%.[21] As shown in table 23, 66.6% of ASCUS smear and 50% of LSIL smear were positive for higher grade lesion. Thus in these cases cytology underestimated lesion severity, hence it is suggested that all ASCUS and LSIL should be subjected to colposcopy, similar suggestion is given by Yarandi F et al.[29] According to Lorincz AT, HPV testing should be done in all ASCUS cases.[30] In 23 cases of unsatisfactory colposcopy, 3 cases were positive on HPR (13.0%), hence it is suggested that all unsatisfactory colposcopy should be consider for ECC where as, in satisfactory colposcopy ECC is not mandatory, similar observation is made by Massad LS.[31]

Low Sensitivity of conventional Pap smear in our study could be due to sampling errors, air-drying effect, or metaplastic maturation of abnormal cells, similar reason reported by Gupta Sodhani S.[32] and Spitzer Mark. [33]

A screening test must be highly sensitive even at the expense of lower specificity.[34] Out of total 316 cases 112 cases were found to be eligible for HPR evaluation, all HPR positive were also diagnosed correctly as positive by colposcopy. Thus overall sensitivity of colposcopy was 100% but the specificity was 20.0% (Table 26).

Table 27 shows correlation of colposcopy diagnosis with histopatholgy results, out of 102 eligible cases for analysis, 46.1% were positive on HPR and 53.9% were negative on HPR. Colposcopy was positive in all HPR positive cases. Where as 80.0% of HPR negative cases were also positive by colposcopy. Thus sensitivity of colposcopy was 100%, where as specificity was only 20.0%, positive predicative value was 51.6% and NPV was 100.00% and diagnostic accuracy was 56.9%.

In low-grade lesion mild acetowhite reaction can be due to HPV infection, immature metaplasia or intraepithelial neoplasia[11], hence resulting in low specificity for low grade lesion. Bharani B, reported colposcopy histopathology correlation is only 30% in low-grade lesion and more in high grade lesion.[22] In our study CIN-1 and CIN-2 cases were over diagnosed on colposcopy. 68.8% of RCI-1 and 37.0% of RCI-2 were reported as chronic cervisitis, on HPR. Mitchell et al selected articles from 1969-1996 and quoted that, the high sensitivity of colposcopy and low specificity in due to **"over calling"** of low-grade lesion, because it is easier to determine that cervix is either normal or very abnormal, than it is to distinguish between minor degree of changes.[11] Reid R, also commented that in BAE (Benign acanthotic epithelium), inflammation, SPI (Sub clinical papilloma infection) can confuse with CIN-1 changes, and are considered as genuine colposcopy errors.[35,36] Elite IM also reported high false positive in CIN-1 by colposcopy.[37]

As shown in table 27, in high grade lesion, sensitivity was 100.0% and specificity was 50.0% In our study, similar observation made by Benedt JL[38] he reported colposcopy sensitivity of 90.3% and specificity of 57.5%. The value of colposcopic impression to identify disease correctly is best with higher the grade of disease predicted (64.2 to 92.6%).[36] Shastri et al from TMH, Mumbai reported colposcopic sensitivity 75.4% and specificity 84.3%.[28] Sundari N, reported colposcopic specificity of 84.6%.[21]

Walker P.G., reported incidence of HPV on cervix 29.0%.[12] In our study HPV was colposcopicaly detected in 6.3% cases and CIN-1 was 15.1%. Our incidence of HPV is low as colposcopicaly CIN-1 and HPV is difficult to differentiate even colposcopy and histology together can not detected all HPV infection, hence colposcopy should be combined with molecular biological studies for HPV.[12]

In our study sensitivity of VIA was 94.1% and specificity was 38.2% (Table 29). Maria Julieta V. Germar, MD in a review article reported range of VIA sensitivity between 49.4%-96%, for specificity between 48.5-97%.[15] Basu PS et al reported sensitivity of 55.7% and specificity 82.1%[39], Sankaranarayanan R. et al in a study from kerela reported sensitivity of 88.6% and specificity of 78.0%.[40] Shashtri et al, reported VIA sensitivity to be 59.7% and specificity 88.4%.[28]

As shown in table 25, follow up of low grade lesion is very important in a women with high risk factors for cancer cervix. In our study (in group-b) 15.9% of RCI-1 lesion progress to RCI-2 inspite of treatment. Cox JT, suggested follow up CIN-1 is necessary as 12% may progress to high grade lesion.[41] Duggan MA et al reported that 18.6% of LSIL progress to CIN-2 and CIN-3[42], Apgar BS and Brotzman Gregory L, reported progression of LSIL to HSIL in 10-20% cases.[43] Melnikow and associate on basis of met analysis in 1998 reported that 47.4% LSIL return to normal, 20.8% progressed to CIN-2 and CIN-3 and 0.15% progress to cancer.[11] In group a none of the lesion advanced (0.0%), 55.5% improved, 34.4% remain same, and 10.3% lost for follow up. As modified RCI scoring method is site specific hence excellent for documentation, follow up and management of low-grade lesion (Table 25).

Parham Groesbeck P, presented a though comparison of cell collection (in vitro) and real time (in vivo) direct visualization technologies used in the screening of women for cervical cancer. Studies using these two approaches have shown to double the detection rate of cervical abnormalities compared with the Pap smear alone and also to decrease the number of false positive results. One of the emerging areas

in cervical cancer is the hypothesis of shedding versus non shedding cervical dysplastic tissue and its role in the false negative Pap smear.[26] Similarly Navratil E, if one considers tremendous value of early diagnosis than colposcopy and cytology together greatly compensates for any error of cytology.[44]

As shown in table 26 out of 102 cases, 46.1% cases which were disease positive on HPR were also correctly diagnosed as positive by colposcopy, where as, as shown in table 27 out of total 98 cases, 48.0% were positive on HPR, but only 46.8% cases were correctly diagnosed by cytology, hence colposcopy diagnosis by modified RCI scoring method was more accurate as compared to cytology this proportion was statically highly significant (P<0.001).

Modified RCI scoring method makes colposcopy diagnosis site specific, therefore very useful in treatment and follow up of low-grade lesions. Time taken is significantly less as compared to conventional method (Table 24). No extra paper work and no extra visits are required. Hence very easy and convenient to both gynaecologist and the women coming to hospital. Considering its very high sensitivity, colposcopy by above method is and ideal screening tool for diagnosis of cancer cervix in secondary and tertiary care teaching hospitals.

SUMMARY AND CONCLUSION

1   After taking clearance from ethical committee, the following study was conducted in the department of obstetrics and gynaecology at NSCB government Medical College, Jabalpur, M.P., India, during 1-9-03 to 30-8-05. Conclusion of this study are based on observation and results.

2   Cervical cancer is the commonest gynaecological cancer of developing countries like India, hence cancer prevention or early detection becomes medico social responsibility and economic necessity. It is quite clear that incidence of cervical cancer can be reduced by appropriate screening, treatment and follow up techniques.

3.   Colposcopy is world wide accepted as most studied and sensitive method for early detection of cancer neoplasia. In spite of this fact, it is not popular method because of interpretive difficulties, inadequate expertise and failure to follow standard diagnostic protocol. To over come above limitation and make colposcopy easy, accurate, economic and time saving , present study was conducted.

4.   In modified RCI scoring method, cervix was divided into four quadrants each quadrant is scored and documented in equation style (Ref. methodology). Main advantage of modified RCI scoring method is, observer variability is minimum, site specification helps in prognosis and follow up of low grade lesions, documentation is less time consuming and self explanatory, hence very good method for teaching and training of colposcopy.

89

5. Majority of women were from urban locality, and 70.2% of them were between 30-50 years of age. Mean age of cases diagnosed as cancer cervix was 47.42±9.83 years and that of RCI-1,RCI-2 and RCI-3 was 35.22±7.87 and 35.68±8.69 and 41.19±10.75 years. This clearly indicates two nodes of age were seen around 35 and 50 years.

6. In present study 96.9% women were multipara and mean age of first coitus was around 16 years, anemia, smoking, low socioeconomic factor, illiteracy were associated co-factors in our study.

7. Majority 96.9% women did not use any barrier method, 65.9% lesion were present on anterior lip of cervix.

8. In present study 83.9% smear were negative of intraepithelial lesion, sensitivity was 46.8% and specificity was 90.2%, 66.6% of ASCUS and 50.0% LSIL cytology were found positive for higher grade lesion on HPR. Hence coloposcopy is mandatory in all ASCUS and LSIL positive smear.

9. A screening test must be highly sensitive even at the expense of lower specificity. In our study overall sensitivity of colposcopy was 100% and specificity was 20.0%. However in high grade lesion sensitivity of colposcopy was 100.0% and specificity was 50.0%.

10 Genuine colposcopy errors are reported in BAE, CIN-1 and SPI cases, as suggested by R. Reid.[33] In our study 68.8% of RCI-1 cases and 37.0% of RCI-2 cases were reported as chronic cervisitis, however in high-grade lesion (RCI-3) colposcopy, histopathology correlation was more than 95.0%.

11. Considering histopathology as gold standard, cytology underestimated diagnosis in 9.0% of CIN-2 cases, 50.0% of CIN-3 cases, 40.0% in CIS, and 50% in SCC cases (Table 23). Proved by various studies including our study, the low sensitivity of cytology warrants the addition of complementary test to maximize sensitivity of cervix cancer screening.

12 By conventional method and mean time required was 19.5±2.4 minutes where as by modified method was significantly less 3.8±1.8 minutes. In conventional method two pages are required per colposcopy record, where as in modified RCI scoring method, no extra pages were required, hence present study is more time saving and economical.

13. With present modification in colposcopy assessment method, reporting becomes simple, quick and easy, for follow up. Treatment of low-grade lesion can be done with confidence (as our method is site specific) hence it is recommended to be implemented in place of conventional colposcopy. Considering very high sensitivity, colposcopy by above method is and ideal screening tool for diagnosis of cancer cervix in secondary and tertiary care teaching hospitals.

BIBLIOGRAPHY

1. Xavier Bosch F., Salvia de Sanjose, Human papiloma virus and cervical cancer. Burden and Assessment of causality, Journal of the National Cancer Institute Monograph no. 31,2003,3-13

2. Thomas E. Rohan, Robert D. Burk and Eduardo L Franco, Towards a reduction of he global burden of cervical cancer. Am J Obstetric Gynecology. 2003, 189 (4): S37-9.

3. Seung Jo Kim, Role of colposcopy and cervicography in the screening and management of precdancerous lesion and early invasive cancer of uterine cervix. J Obstetric Gynecology of India. 2000, 50(5): 134-46.

4. Sankaranarayan R., C. Mahe, cervical cancer control in the developing world. Ind. J of Gynecologic oncology. 2004, 4(2):5-13.

5. Saranath D., Notani Perin, human papilloma viruses and cervical cancer. Bulletin of the Jaslok Hospital and Research Center. 2004, 28(4): 1-18.

6. ACOG committee on practice Bulletins. ACOG Practice bulletins: Clinical management guidelines for Obstetrics gynecologist. Number 45, August 2003. Cervical Cytology screening (replaces committee opinion 152, March 1995) Obstet gyneacol, 2003 Aug: 102(2): 417-27.

7. Wright V. Cecil, MD, FRCS(C), understanding the colposcope, contemporary colposcopy obstetrics and gynecology clinics of north America, ISSN-0889-8545, March 1993, Vol. 20 (1):31-46.

8. Saraiya U., Das S.K., Nigam Sudha, Batra Aruna, Chandra Mithilesh, Diagnostic problems and limitation of colposcopy cytology, An atlas of colposcopy, cytology and histopathology of lower female genital tract, 19th edition, 1995, CBS publishers: 110-117.

9. Sellors John W, Mieminen Pekka, Vesterinen Erov and Pavonen Jorma. Observer variability in the scoring of colpophotographs. Obstetrics and gynecology. 1990, 76(6): 1006-8.

10 Sellors JohnW, Sankarnarayanan R., An introduction to CIN,colposcopy and treatment of CIN, A Beginners mannual, IARC, Lyon 2003: 13-19.

11 Mitchell D. Greenberg, "Reids Colpocopic Index" in Colposcopy Principles and Practice, an Intergrated Text Book and Atlas. WB Saunders Company, Philadelphia, USA, 2002: 213-224.

12 Walker P.G., Singer A., Dyson J.L., Shah K.V., Wilters J. and Coleman D.V., Colposcopy in the diagnosis of papilloma virus infection of the uterine cervix, British Journal of obstetric Gynecology, Vol. 99, Nov. 1983: 1982-1086.

13 Monsonego J. Colposcopy : The value of HPV testing in clinical practice, Gynaecol Obstet fertil, 2004 Jan; 32(1): 62-74.

14 YuBK, Kuo BI etal, Improved early detection of cervical intraepithelial lesion by combination of conventional pap smear and speculo scopy, Eur J. Gynaecol Oncol, 2003;24(6): 495-9.

15 Julieta V Maria, Germar M.D., Visual Inspection with acetic acid as a cervical cancer screening tool for developing countries. http://www.gfmer.ch/Endo/course 2003/visual inspection cervical_cancer.htm accessed on 9/22/2004.

16 Das S.K., Suri S. et al, Colposcopy and new adjunctive methods for cervical cancer screening, frontiers in obstetrics and gynecology, Jaypee publication 2nd edition, 1999: 289-296.

17 Etherington IJ, Dun J. Shafi MI, Smith T, Luesley DM, video Colpography; a new technique for secondary cervical screening, Br. J Obstetric Gynecology, 1997 Jun; 104(6): 718-27.

18 Charvet I, Meda P, Genet M. Pette MF, Viastosat. Optical diagnosis of cervical dysplasia, Bull Cancer, 2004 Jan; 91(1): 45-53.

19 Bhatt Rohit , preventive gynaecological oncology, obs. & gynee today, Feb 2003,Vol. VIII(2): 66-73.

20 Buxton E.J., Luesley D.M., Shafi M.I., Rollason M. Colposcopically directed punch biopsy: a potentially misleading investigation,BJOG,Dec. 1991,Vol. 98: 1273-1276.

21 Sundari N., Prevalence of CIN in urban population: Role of screening colposcopy, Asian Journal of Obst & Gyn. practice, March 2002,Vol. 4(2): 16-19.

22 Bharani B, Phatak S. Role of colposcopy in evaluation of lower female genital tract in 175 symptomatic women. J. Obstetric Gynaecology, India, 2004, 54 (4): 372-75.

23 Bhatla N., Tumours of the cervix uteri, Jeffcoate's principles of gynaecology. International edition, Arnold publishers, London, 338 Euston road, NW 13BH, 2001: 444-465.

24 WHO (1986) Control of Cancer of cervix uteri, A WHO meeting bulletin of WHO 1986, 64: 607-18.

25 Disaia Philip J, William Creasman T, preinvasive disease of the cervix. Clinical gynaecologic oncology, fith edition publication Mosby,1997: 1-32

26 Kenneth B, Hatch, Jonathan Bereck S, Intraepithelial disease of cervix, vagina and valva chapter 16, Novak's text book of gynaecology Lepincott williams and wilkins 2002: 471-480

27 Disaia Philp J, MD, Shedding a new light on Bethesda III: New technologies in cervical screening, Am J Obstetric Gynaecology, Vol. 188, 2003, No-3, S1-S5.

28 Shastri SS, Dinshaw K, Amin G, Gosswami S, Chinoy R, Kane S, Kelkar R, et al, concurrent evaluation of visual, cytological and HPV testing as scrrening method for the early detection of cervical neoplasia in TMH Mumbai, India, Bull world health org, March 2005,Vol. 83(3): 186-194.

29 Yarandi F., Izadi Mood N., Mirahafi, Eftekhar Z, colposcopic and histologic findings in women with a cytologic dianosis of a typical squamous cells of undermined significance; Aust-NZJ Obstet. Gynecol. 2004 Dec; 44(6): 524-6.

30 Lorincz AT, Screening for cervical cancer: new alternatives and research. Sal publica Mex, 2003; 45 Suppl 3: S376-87.

31   Massad LS, Collins YC, using history and colposcopy to select women for endocervical curettage. Results from 2,287 cases, J Repod Med, 2003 Jan, 48(1): 1-6.

32   Gupta S, Sodhani P. Why is high-grade squamous intraepithelial neoplasia under diagnosed on cytology in a quarter of case ? Analysis of smear character tics in discrepant cases, Indian J Cancer, 2004, Jul-Sep: 41(3): 104-8.

33   Mark Spitzer, M.D, and Cervical screening adjuncts: Recent advances AJOG review, AMJ. Obstetric. Gynecology, 1998, Vol. 179, No. 2: 544-556.

34   Jacqueline D. Sherris, cervical cancer prevention; A strategic opportunity to improve womens reproductive health, International family planning perspectives, Jan. 1999 Vol. 25. http/www.agi_usa.org/pubs/journals/25s5699.html.

35   Reid R, M.B., B.S.C., Robert Stanhope, Barry, Herschman,et al, Genital warts and cervical cancer, a colposcopic index for differentiating sub clinical papillomaviral infection from cervical intraepithelial neoplasia, Am J Obstetric. Gynecology, August 15, 1984,Vol.149(8): 815-823.

36   Richard Reid, Barry R., Herschman, Cristopher P., Crum., Yaoshi Fu, Lundy Braun, Keerti, V. Shah et al, Genital warts and cervical cancer The tissue basis of colposcopic change, Am J. Obstetric Gynaecolgy. June 1,1984,Vol.149(5):293-301.

37   Elite IM. Pitfalls in the diagnosis of cervical intra epithelial neoplasia 1, J. Low Genityract Dis 2004 Jul; 8(3): 18-17, http://www.ncbi.nlm.nih.gov/entrez/query.fcgi?cmd.6/17/05.

38 Benedet J.L., Anderson GH, MB and B.A. Boyes, Colposcopic accuracy in the diagnosis of micro invasive and occult Invasive Carcinoma of the Cervix. April 1985Vol. 65, No. 4: 557-562.

39 Basu PS, Sankar narayanan R, Mandal R, Roy C, Das P. Choudhary D et al Visual inspection with acetic acid and cytology in the early detection of cervical neoplasia in Kolkatta, India, Int. J. Gynecol.cancer, Sept.-Oct. 2003, Vol.13(5):   626-632

40 Sankar narayanan R, Wesley R, Thara S. Dhakad N., etal Test Characteristics of visual inspection with 4% acetic acid (VIA) and lugol's iodine (VILI) in cervical cancer screening in Kerela, India, Int. J. Gynecol. Cancer. Sep-Oct 2003,Vol. 106(3):   404-408.

41 Cox JT. Schiffman M, Solomon D: ASCUS-LSIL triage study ATLS group, Am J obstet gynecol, June 2003,Vol. 188(6): 1406-1412.

42 Duggan MA, Mc Gregor SE, Stuart GC et al, The natural history of cervical human papilloma virus (HPV) infections based on prospective follow up, Br. J Obstet Gynaecol, 1985,92; 1086.

43 Apgar BS., Gregory L. Brotzman, high grade squamaus intra epithelial lesion, Chapter 11, colposcopy prinicipes and practice, An Integrated Text book and atlas, W.B. Saunders company, 2002: 249-263.

44 Navratil E, Burghardt E., Bajardi F., Graz. Austria, and W. Nash, New York, Simutaneous colposcopy and cytology used in screening for carcinoma of the cervix, Am J Obst. And Gynaecology. June 1958, Vol. 75(6): 1293-1296.

"COLPOSCOPIC ASSESSMENT BY MODIFIED RCI SCROING METHOD IN DETECTION OF CERVICAL LESIONS"

DR. KAVITA N. SINGH

Name..Reg.............................

Address...Age in year's.................

1. Area ☐

   1. Urban   2. Rural

2. Marital Status ☐

   1. Married   2. Widow   3. Divorcee 4. Single

3. Occupation

(A)   **Husband** ☐

   1. Labourer   2. Farmer   3. Business 4. Service   5. Driver

(B)   **Wife** ☐

   1. Labourer   2. Housewife 3. Others

4. Age of first Sexual Contact (in years) ☐

   1. < 15 Years   2.   > 15-16 Years   3.   > 16-17 Years

   4. > 17-18 Years   5.   > 18 Years

5. Complaints ☐

   1.   While Discharge   2.   Irreguler Bleeding P/V

   3.   Postcoital Spotting   4.   Itching

   5.   Pain in abdomen   6.   Burning Micturition

   7.   No Complaints

6. Parity ☐

   1. P_0 2. P_2 3. P_2 4. P_3 5. P_4 6. P_5

   7. P_6 & Above -7

7. Abortion ☐

1. A_0 2. A_1 3. A_2 4. A_3 5. $>A_3$

8. History of Contraceptive Used ☐

1. Nil   2. Condoms   3. OC's

4. TT/VT   5. Injection   6. Others

9. History of Medical Illness ☐

1. Diabetics   2. HT   3. TB   4. Anaemia   5. Others

10. History of treatment of lower genital tract ☐

(A) 1. Once   2. Twice   3. Thrice

(B) 1. Medical   2. Surgical

11. P/S Examination ☐

1. Healthy Ex,vagina but cytology abnormal 2. Infection   3. Errosion

4. Hypertrophied   5.NF   6. Old tear   7. Others

12. Associated Gyn. Condition ☐

1. Normal uterus   2. Bully/MPS/Adenomyosis 3. Fibroid   4. PID

4. DUB   6. Others

13. Colposcopy Form

VIA ☐

1. Positive   2. Negative   3. Inconclusive

14. VIAM ☐

   1. Positive   2. Negative   3. Inconclusive

15. VILI ☐

   1. Positive   2. Negative   3. Inconclusive

16. Colposcopy Findings ☐

1. **Normal**

2. **Abnormal Colposcopy Finding**

(a) Within T Z   ☐☐☐☐   (b) Outside TZ (Ex. -Ectocx, Vagina etc) ☐☐☐☐

(1) AW   (1) AW
(2) Flat   (2) Flat
(3) PN   (3) PN
(4) MO   (4) MO
(5) Keratosis   (5) Keratosis
(6) Iodine-Ve   (6) Iodine-Ve
(7) Micropapillary or Microconvoluted   (7)Micropapillary or Microconvoluted
(8) AV   (8) AV

17. RCI Score ☐

1. 0-2   2. 3-4   3. 5-8

18. ☐

4. LU   1. RU

3. LL   2. RL

19. Colposcopically Suspected Invasive Ca. ☐

1. Yes   2. No

20. Unsatisfactory Colposcopy ☐

1. Yes   2. No

21. Misc Finding ....

....

22. Biopsy taken ☐

(1) Yes   (2) No

23. Paps Report (Bethesda system) □

(1) WNL

(2) **Benign Cellular changes** □

(1) TV   (2) Reactive Changes to Inflamm.

(3) Associated with infection   (4) Atrophy with Inflammation

(3) **Epithelial Cell abrormolities** □

(1) ASCUS   (2) Glandular cell

(3) LSIL   (a) Benign   (b) Malignant

(4) HSIL   (5) Sq. Cell Ca.

(6) Other Malig.

24. Colposcopy Diagnosis : ....

25. Cytology Diagnosis : ....

26. Biopsy Diagnosis : ....

27. Final Impression □

(1) Low grade CIN   (2) High grade CIN

(3) Invasive Carcinoma   (4) Condyloma Accuminata

(5) Ectorpion   (6) Sq. Metaplasia

(7) Endo Cervical polyp   (8) Others

28. Remarks : ....

: ....

APPENDIX-B

Preparation of 5% acetic acid, Lugol's iodine soulution, and Monsel's paste

5% dilute acetic acid

Ingredients	Quantity
1. Glacial acetic acid	5 ml
2. Distilled water	95 ml

Preparation

Cerefully and 5ml of glacial acetic acid into 95ml of distilled water and mix thoroughly.

Storage :

Unused acetic acid should be discarded at the end of the day.

Label :

5% dilute acetic acid

Note : It is important to remember to dilute the glacial acetic acid, since the undiluted strength causes a severe chemical burn if applied to the epithelium.

Lugol's iodine solution

Ingredients	Quantity
1. Postassium iodide	19 g
2. Distilled water	100 ml
3. Iodine crystals	5 g

Preparation

A. Dissolve 10g postassium iodide in 100 ml of distilled water.

B. Slowly add 5 g iodine crystals, while shaking.

C. Filter and store in tightly stoppered brown bottle.

Storage :

1 month

Label :

Lugol's iodine solution

Use by (date)

APPENDIX-C

Table - Reid's Colposcopic Index[11]

Colposcopic	0 Point	1 Point	2 Point
Margin	Condylomatous or micropapillary contour Indistinct borders, Flocculated or feathered, Jagged, angular , satelite lesion, aw beyond TZ.	Regular lesion with smooth, Sharp margins	rolled, peeling edges
Color	Shiny, snow-white, semitransparent, opaque	shiny, gray-white intermediate white	Dull, oyster gray
Vessels	Uniform, fine caliber Nondilated capilary loops fine punctation or mosaic	Absence of surface Vessels vessels dilated.	Definite punctuation or mosaic individual
Iodine staining	positive iodine uptake	partial iodine uptake lesion.	Yellow staining of
Colposcopic Score	0-2=HPV or CIN-1	3-4=CIN 1 or CIN2	5-8 = CIN2 or CIN3

APPENDIX-D

INTERNATIONAL COLPOSCOPIC TERMINOLOGY[7]

Normal colposcopic findings
    Original squamous epithelium
    Columnar epithelium
    Normal transformation zone
Abnormal colposcopic findings
    Within the transformation zone
      Acetowhite epithelium*
      Flat
      Micropapillary or microconvoluted
      Punctation*
      Mosaic*
      Leukoplakia*
      Iodine negative
      Atypical vessels
Outside the transformation zone, e.g.,
      ectocervix, vagina
      Acetowhite epithelium*
      Micropapillary or microconvoluted
      Punctation*
      Mosaic*
      Leukoplakia*
      Iodine negative
      Atypical vessels

Coposcopically suspect invasive
carcinoma
Unsatisfactory colposcopy
    Squamocolumnar juction not visible
    Severe inflammation or severe atrophy
    Cervix not visible

Miscellaneous findings
    Nonacetowhite micropapillary surface
    Exophytic condyloma
    Inflammation
    Ulcer
    Other

*Indicates minor or major changes: Minor changes = acetowhite epithelium, fine mosaic, fine punctation, and thin leukoplakia. Major changes = dense acetowhite epithelium, coarse mosaic, coarse puncation, thick leukoplakia, atypical vessels, and erosion.

Ratified by the International Federation of Cervical Pathology and Colposcopy, May 1990, Rome, Italy.

The transformation zone is the origin of intraepithelial lesions of the cervix and thus forms the basis of the classification system. The International Federation of Cervical Pathology and Colposcopy (IFCPC) has formulated the classification system as shown in above table. This system includes lesions extending outside the transformation zone as not uncommonly seen with papillomavirus infection, although their neoplastic potential is small.

APPENDIX-E

THE 2001 BETHESDA SYSTEM : REPORTING CATEGORIES[10]

Negative for intraepithelial lesion or malignancy

Epithelial cell abnormalities

   Squamous cell

      Atypical squamous cell (ASC)

      'of undetermined significance' (ASC-US)

      'cannot exclude HSIL' (ASC-H)

   Low-grade squamous intraepithelial lesion (LSIL)

   High-grade squamous intraepithelial lesion (HSIL)

   Squamous Cell carcinoma

   Glandular

      Atypical glandular cells (AGC)

      (specify endocervical, endometrial, or not otherwise specified)

      Atypical glandular cells, favour neoplastic (specify endocervical, or not otherwise specified)

      Endocervical adenocarcinoma in situ (AIS)

      Adenocarcinoma

   Other (list not comprehensive)

   Endometrial cells in a woman over 40 years of age

APPENDIX-F

CONVENTIONAL COLPOSCOPY RECORD[10]

1. Medical Record Number: _____

2. Patient's Name: _____

3. Age: _____

4. Date of visit: _____ / _____ / _____ (Day/Month/Year)

5. Colposcopist performing exam : _____

6. Did you see the entire squamocolumnar juction (SCJ)?   Yes   No
   (If 'No', consider endocervical curettage)

7. Unsatisfactory colposcopy:

   ☐ Entire SCJ not visualised   ☐ Entire lesion not visualised

8. Colposcopic findings within the transformation zone (use √ to indicate result):
   (Draw SCJ, acetowhite, punctation, mosaics, atypical vessels, and other lesions)

   ☐ Flat acetowhite epithelium

   ☐ Micropapillary or microconvoluted acetowhite epithelium

   ☐ Leukoplakia

   ☐ Punctation

   ☐ Mosaic

   ☐ Atypecal vessels

   ☐ Iodine-negative epithelium

   ☐ Other, specify: _____

9. Findings outside the transformation zone: _____

_____

10. Colposcopically suspect invasive carcinoma :   Yes   No

11. Miscellaneous findings: _____

107

12. Colposcopic diagnosis (use ☐ to indicate result) :

    ☐   Unsatisfactory, specify:

    ☐   Normal colposcopic findings

    ☐   Inflammation/infection, specify:

    ☐   Leukoplakia

    ☐   Condyloma

    ☐   Low-grade CIN

    ☐   High-grade CIN

    ☐   Invasive cancer, specify location referral: _____

    ☐   Other, specify: _____

    ☐   Number of biopsies taken _____ (mark site(s) with an 'X' on colposcopy drawing)

    ☐   Endocervical curettage (ECC) taken

13. Other findings (use to indicate all that apply):

    ☐   Lesion extended into endocervix

    ☐   Mucosal bleeding easily induced

    ☐   Purulent cervicitis

    ☐   Opaque discharge

    ☐   Yellow discharge

    ☐   Other, specify: _____

14. Colposcopist's signature: _____

15. If test performed at colposcopy exam, note results below:

lgefr & i=

uke & ---
---------- mez---
irk & --
--------- fnukad --

eSa nwjchu i)fr dkYiksLdksih }kjk van:uh tkWp djokus ds fy;s rS;kj gwW] eq>s bl izfdz;k dh iwjh tkudkjh] tkWp ls ykHk o ijs'kkfu;kW   MkWDVj--------------------
----------------------}kjk le>k nh xbZ gS A vko';drk gksus ij ck;ksIlh (Biopsy) ds fy;s Hkh eSa rS;kj gwW A tkWp ls cPpknkuh eq[k ds dSalj dh 'kq:vkr gksus dk tYnh irk py tkrk gS A ;g ,d 'kks/k dk fo"k; gS] ;g eq>s crk fn;k x;k gS A eq>s fdlh izdkj dh dksbZ Hkh vkifRr ugh gS A eSa mijksDr tkWo o bykt ds fy;s iw.kZr% lger gwW A

xokg %   gLrk{kj

APPENDIX-H

ABBREVIATION

AIS	Adenocarcinoma in situ
ASCUS	Atypical squamous cells of undetermined significance
BAE	Benign acanthotic epithelium
CIN	Cervical intraepithelial neoplasia
CIS	Carcinoma in situ
CM	Centimeter
ECC	Endocervical curettage
HPV	Human papillomavirus
HSIL	High grade squamous intraepithelial lesion
IEL	Intraepithelial lesion
LSIL	Low grade squamous intraepithelial lesion
NF	Nabothian follicle
OC's	Oral Contraceptives
OPD	Out patient deparment
PS	Per speculum
RCI	Reid colposcopic index
SCJ	Squamo columnar junction
SIL	Squamous intraepithelial lesion
SPI	Subclinical papilloma infection
SCC	Squamous cell carcinoma
TBS	Terminology Bethesda System
TZ	Transformation Zone
VIA	Visual inspection with acetic acid
VILI	Visual inspection with Lugol's iodine
WHO	World Health Organization
WNL	Within normal limit

 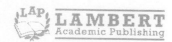 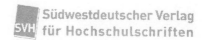